How To Survive In a World Without Antibiotics

by Keith Scott-Mumby MD, MB ChB, PhD

Scott-Mumby Wellness

PO Box 19452,
Reno, Nevada, USA
email: scottmumbywellness@gmail.com

How To Survive In a World Without Antibiotics

ISBN-13: 978-0983878421

Library of Congress: this work is acknowledged by the Library of Congress, with dated receipt and is therefore fully protected. We are awaiting a registration number, which will be affixed to subsequent print runs.

Printed in USA by CreateSpace

Cover design and layout by Dragos Balasoiu - www.dragosb.com/design

Disclaimer

Title Quote

Put bluntly, medicine's successes at vaccination and antibiotics treatment are trivial accomplishments relative to natural selection's success at generating the immune system. Recognizing this fact has important repercussions for the long-term control of infectious diseases. We will probably obtain better disease control by figuring out how to further tweak the immune system and capitalize on its vastly superior abilities than by relying on some human intervention such as new antimicrobials (antibiotics, antivirals, or antoprotozoal agents).

Paul W. Ewald Plague Time

Quotes And Facts

The mass of a single cell of the E coli bacterium is 665 femtograms. A femtogram is one-thousandth of a picogram, which is one-thousandth of a nanogram, which is a billionth of a gram.

Journal of Applied Physics.

....

Not only does the Earth contain more bacterial organisms than all others combined (scarcely surprising, given their minimal size and mass); not only do bacteria live in more places and work in a greater variety of metabolic ways; not only did bacteria alone constitute the first half of life's history, with no slackening in diversity thereafter; but also, and most surprisingly, total bacterial biomass (even at such minimal weight per cell) may exceed all the rest of life combined, even forest trees, once we include the subterranean populations as well.

Stephen Jay Gould, "Planet of the Bacteria," Washington Post Horizon, 1996, 119 (344): H1; Reprinted here with permission; This essay was adapted from Full House, New York: Harmony Books, 1996, pp. 175-192.

....

Bacteria inhabit effectively every place suitable for the existence of life. Mother told you, after all, that bacterial "germs" require constant vigilance to combat their ubiquity in every breath and every mouthful, and the vast majority of bacteria are benign or irrelevant to us, not harmful agents of disease. One fact will suffice: during the course of life, the number of E. coli in the gut of each human being far exceeds the total number of people that now live and have ever lived.

Stephen Jay Gould, "Planet of the Bacteria," Washington Post Horizon, 1996, 119 (344): H1; Reprinted here with permission; This essay was adapted from Full House, New York: Harmony Books, 1996, pp. 175-192.

....

Numerical estimates, admittedly imprecise, are a stock in trade of all popular writing on bacteria. The Encyclopaedia Britannica tells us that bacteria live by "billions in a gram of rich garden soil and millions in one drop of saliva." Human skin harbors some 100,000 microbes per square centimeter (note:

"microbes" in-cludes nonbacterial unicells, but the overwhelming majority of "microbes" are bacteria).

Writer Dorion Sagan and biologist Lynn Margulis, Garden of Microbial Delights

Fully 10 percent of our own dry body weight consists of bacteria, some of which, although they are not a congenital part of our bodies, we can't live without.

Writer Dorion Sagan and biologist Lynn Margulis, Garden of Microbial Delights

We could not digest and absorb food properly without our gut "flora." Grazing animals, cattle and their relatives, depend upon bacteria in their stomachs to digest grasses in the process of rumination. About 30 percent of atmospheric methane can be traced to the action of methanogenic bacteria in the guts of ruminants, largely released into the atmosphere—how else to say it—by belches and farts.

Stephen Jay Gould, "Planet of the Bacteria," Washington Post Horizon, 1996, 119 (344): H1; Reprinted here with permission; This essay was adapted from Full House, New York: Harmony Books, 1996, pp. 175-192.

In another symbiosis essential to human agriculture, plants need nitrogen as an essential soil nutrient but cannot use the ubiquitous free nitrogen of our atmosphere. This nitrogen is "fixed," or chemically converted into usable form, by the action of bacteria like Rhizobium, living symbiotically in bulbous growths on the roots of leguminous plants.

Stephen Jay Gould, "Planet of the Bacteria," Washington Post Horizon, 1996, 119 (344): H1; Reprinted here with permission; This essay was adapted from Full House, New York: Harmony Books, 1996, pp. 175-192.

A group, led by microbiologist William. B. Whitman, estimates the total number of bacteria on Earth to be five million trillion trillion -- that's a five with 30 zeroes after it. Look at it this way. If each bacterium were a penny, the stack would reach a trillion light years. These almost incomprehensible numbers give only a sketch of the vast pervasiveness of bacteria in the natural world. "There simply hadn't been any estimates of the number of bacteria on Earth," said Whitman. "Because they are so diverse and important, we thought it made sense to get a picture of their magnitude."

The study was published in the June 1998 Proceedings of the National Academy of Sciences.

....

For the first half of geological time our ancestors were bacteria. Most creatures still are bacteria, and each one of our trillions of cells is a colony of bacteria.

Richard Dawkins

....

"Love: Before I heard the doctors tell The dangers of a kiss; I had considered kissing you. The nearest thing to bliss. But now I know biology and sit and sigh and moan; six million mad bacteria and I thought we were alone!"

Song lyrics

....

A probe sent two miles underground in a South American gold mine found bacteria living there. Their dinner? Radioactive emissions from the rocks around them. Above ground, the aptly named Deinococcus radiodurans can handle radiation exposure nearly 10,000 times the fatal dose for humans.

Somewhere in cyberspace...

....

Everything we do with food is an attempt to keep from being poisoned by our microbial competitors.

Professor Paul Sherman, Cornell University.

Contents

Appendix

Terminology

Let's just go over a few terms so that when you meet them you will be clear about the meaning.

Antibiotic: means a substance which will KILL bacteria and similar organisms (but not viruses).

Viricidal: A substance which will kill viruses (but not bacteria).

Bacteriostatic: means a substance which will handicap bacteria, by preventing them growing and multiplying. It does not actually kill bacteria but holds them in check, while the person's immune system gets to work, mopping up the invader.

Antiseptic: A substance (or process, like UV light) which kills all living organisms on a surface. In reality most antiseptics will kill 95% or more. But nothing is ever 100%.

Hygienic: Germs reduced to a level where the body is not at risk.

Sterile: No surviving viable germs of any kind.

MRSA... What's all the fuss?

MRSA (pronounced "mersa") is an abbreviation for "methicillin-resistant Staphylococcus aureus", the hospital superbug. Staph. aureus is a common bacteria but certain strains have become resistant to almost all known antibiotics, including powerful modern penicillins (such as methicillin). Today, methicillin is no longer made and has been replaced by newer variants, such as oxacillin, flucloxacillin and dicloxacillin.

It has raised extreme concern, not because of its own damaging powers (which are not inconsiderable), but because it is seen as the flagship of worse to come. As you will read, antibiotic-resistant bacteria have been around almost from the beginning of the "antibiotic era". But something about the MRSA problem makes it clear that we have come to the end of a golden age of healthcare, where infectious disease were seen to be only an occasional or trivial problem. Those who chanced to die of an infection were seen as just "unlucky".

We no longer fear pneumonia, bacterial endocarditis, brain abcesses, and other terrible conditions that swept away our loved ones in a matter of days. We have become complacent. It's been a great period in which to live. I was born in 1945, just as antibiotics hit the market. We have lost nobody in my family due to infections in the years since!

But we will soon return to the days when antibiotics are of little help. People will die in huge numbers, unless they take the trouble to learn the alternatives. The irony is, as I keep saying, that there are hundreds of alternatives. But arrogant colleagues sneer at these, as if they were just old wives' tales and superstitions.

In fact the real folly and superstition has been mainstream medicine, which has continued to believe in the silly fairy tale of endless life with antibiotics. I repeat: the threat of resistance has been there right from the start. They just ignored it.

Now you are lucky, you can re-learn about the old remedies, which really worked. But I'm going to give you the science too, lots of science and studies, which show this is no folklore but perfectly genuine and humble remedies, which are easy to self-administer and cost very little to obtain or make.

I'm sorry to do this, in a way, but I need to raise your concern level so that you understand how critical this is. Take a look at this picture, which is a man's leg after surgery to clean up an infection of "flesh eating bacteria". You can see how it got that name. Cutting away his infected skin and tissues was the only way to save his life, when antibiotics no longer work.

There's worse still at the end of section 28. Please! I urge you, take the end of antibiotics as something very serious.

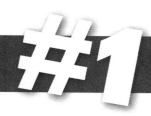

MRSA "fever" struck the country with the publication of a telling article in the Journal of the American Medical Association (JAMA 17th Oct 2007). That morning I was invited on a radio show to discuss the problem and get it into perspective. I had recently published an article likening the community active form of MRSA (as opposed to the hospital "superbug" version) to the Black Death from ages past.

One of the other guests, who I suppose I should not name, was being interviewed by several radio stations, including the one I was on. He blamed illegal immigrants, claiming it was their dirty habits and lack of personal responsibility that had caused the problem; he also blamed foreigners for tape worms, TB, Chagas' disease and a whole host of other dangerous health conditions.

I followed him and declared his opinion "fascist, unscientific, irrational and inciting prejudice and hatred". Fortunately, he had left to spread his poison somewhere else by the time I said this, otherwise a war of bitter words would have broken out. No matter, I stand by my condemnation of this foolish and ignorant tirade. It's akin to hysteria. The studio presenter, normally a very mild and civilized man, ended up raising his voice in shock at what "these people are doing to our country".

This is how mob violence gets started.

The presenter only calmed down when I pointed out the stupidity of blaming foreigners, when Americans travel overseas and are just as capable of bringing back pathogens as newcomers! And what about legal immigrants? Does he suppose that bacteria have a way of knowing who's legal and who isn't?

I myself contracted Cholera while working on my 2004 Tsunami rescue mission to Sri Lanka and brought that to Pasadena (much to the shock of the public health officials):

http://www.scott-mumby.com/mission1.html

I was not an illegal alien.

As to the tapeworm, that was just pig ignorance (slight pun intended!) Parasites have been endemic in the US, especially the Deep South, for centuries. Transmission is by food and from pets, rarely by direct human contact. There are some bad beasties here, as you will know if you have

visited my parasite page: http://www.alternative-doctor.com/allergies/
parasites.htm

For example, 25- 30% of the population of the south-eastern USA, mainly
children, have whip worm (Trichuris species) and my textbook sources are
impeccable: *(Schmidt GD, Roberts LS, Foundations of Parasitology, Times
Mirror/Mosby College Publishing, St. Louis, 1989, p. 418).*

Ironically, I might be warning healthy Europeans to take care when they
come to the USA!

So with the political frenzy disposed of, what do we know?

MRSA was actually caused by doctors, not immigrants. It's an inevitable
result of overuse of antibiotics, followed by tougher strains of penicillin (like
methicillin), used to try and clean up the stubborn bugs, and the eventual
emergence of resistance even to methicillin.

It's uncertain what the true incidence is because it is not at this time a
notifiable disease. But the 2008 JAMA article worked by extrapolating from
earlier 2005 figures and is, in effect, a mere guess. There were 5,287
invasive infections reported that year in the regions studied, which would
translate to an estimated 94,360 cases nationally. There were 988 reported
deaths among infected people in the study; around 20% and this was simply
extrapolated up to 18,650.

IF THE STUDY FIGURES ARE CORRECT — and I emphasize they are only an
intelligent guess, which I accept as such — then MRSA is killing more people
than AIDS. 988 out of 94,360 cases gives a rate of 6.3 per 100,000. That
would translate to 18,650 deaths annually (the researchers admit they don't
even know if MRSA was the cause in all cases). AIDS killed an estimated
17,011 Americans in 2005.

Scare Talk? I don't think so

You might think this is scare talk' "Of course this thing will never get out of control". You are wrong. It is already out of control. The unanswered question is will it spread like wildfire, or just continue as a grumbling danger lurking below the surface?

Let's just hope that the pandemic model won't happen. As I said there are strong parallels with the Medieval "Black Death" but microbial disease is just not predictable. The important point to keep in mind is that pandemic infections, like any other infection, are NOT caused just by pathogenic microbes.

Infectious disease is caused by a lowered immune system. Period.

Healthy individuals, with a vibrant immune system and a positive mental attitude will not succumb to pathogens, no matter how vicious they are. I lived in a malarious country for years, with no prophylaxis, got bitten a dozen times a day by mosquitoes and caught nothing (there was even dengue fever present in our city).

We are in balance with Nature. She has invented NOTHING we cannot handle, if our defence mechanisms are working properly. Always remember that; it's important. But disease gets started because individuals are weakened by negative factors, such as overload, malnutrition, shock and stress. If we avoid these factors, or correct them quickly, there is no reason to fear disease.

Be healthy, that's your best protection. Remember my #1 motto is this: any good health measure is an anti-infection measure (same with cancer).

If you are struck down in a pandemic of any kind, you can forget the idea that the doctor will come along and help you. Even if the medical profession knew how to deal with such a problem, which it doesn't, there would simply not be enough doctors to go around. You will be on your own.

You need to read this report carefully and NEVER throw it away.

How many valiant men, how many fair ladies, breakfast with their kinfolk and the same night supped with their ancestors in the next world! The condition of the people was pitiable to behold. They sickened by the thousands daily, and died unattended and without help. Many died in the open street, others dying in their houses, made it known by the stench of their rotting bodies. Consecrated churchyards did not suffice for the burial of the vast multitude of bodies, which were heaped by the hundreds in vast trenches, like goods in a ships hold and covered with a little earth.

Giovanni Boccaccio

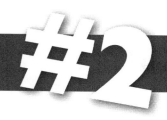

Bacteria are single-celled organisms. They come in a variety of shapes: round spheres (called a coccus, plural cocci), rod-shaped (called a bacillus, plural bacilli), spiral- shaped (called a spirochete, plural spirochetes) and a few odd-balls (no plural!)

Bacteria are the oldest living organisms on planet Earth. Since they don't produce "babies" (offspring), but reproduce by just splitting in two, you could say that bacteria represent an original founding organism which is now billions of years old!

Estimates of how many cells make up a human being vary—between 1 trillion and 100 trillion. I've seen both.

But what is clear is that there are 10 TIMES more bacteria in you and on you than the actual number of cells that go to make up YOU!

You are about 10% dry weight of bacteria: that's you, your body and your cells, minus the water in your tissues.

If you took away all the connective tisues of a human being, just leaving the cells, you'd have the equivalent of 9 human beings in your gut, so far as cell numbers were concerned; THAT'S how big a deal bacteria are for us.

Bacteria have only one single strand of DNA that encodes their nature. We humans have about 25,000- 30,000 genes that make up our humanness.

But there are over 100 times more bacterial genes, on you and in you, which all that matters. That's 3 million genes, set against your measly 1%. **What happens to your bacteria, happens to you. Trust me.**

We need lots of respect for those single-cell organisms that are all-but part of us. In fact bacteria keep us alive. The friendly ones act like body armour and prevent pathogenic invaders from destroying us. They keep the outer environment under control, so we stay healthy. They digest our food. They make certain vitamins for us.

Remember, the vast majority of bacteria are friendly or at least harmless. There are just a few troublemakers that create disease and death.

However, there is a real mystery. How do they do anything at all? I mean, there is no brain or nervous system. They don't have any obvious means of communicating or interacting. How do bacteria get organized to make somebody sick or healthy? They are so tiny and inconsequential, it seems unreasonable they could affect us at all, while acting individually.

Well, according to Professor Bonnie Bassler at Princeton there has been a breakthrough discovery. Bacteria, it seems, have a secret chemical conversation system. It's called "quorum sensing." As it turns out, every type of bacteria makes and secretes small molecules (a bit like hormones). When a bacterium is alone, these molecules have no effect (no receptors).

But when there's a large enough group of bacteria, these secreted molecules reach a critical level and suddenly all the bacteria begin to act as a synchronized group, based on the characteristic behavior programmed into the genes.

This was first discovered by Bassler, observing a marine bacterium called Vibrio fischeri. This little organism emits light. But when a suspension of bacteria is so dilute they are, in effect, isolated, nothing happens. Only when the bacterial concentration—and hence the level of quorum sensing signals—reaches a certain level, then all the bacteria "switch on" at once and begin to glow in the dark. It seems remarkable that tiny organelles, without any apparent sense organs, can suddenly tell who is in the neighborhood and how many neighbors there are!

Incidentally, they can talk inter-species too. A second quorum sensing mechanism, possessed of all bacteria and working interspecies, is what Bassler calls a "bacterial Esperanto".

The implications of this are devastating. Consider a pathogenic organism inside your body. If a few bacteria released their virulence, it would have no effect. You are at least a trillion times bigger than they are.

But they grow and multiply and when their quorum sensing tells them there are enough cronies present, they all launch their virulence attack at the same time. This way they are able to suddenly overwhelm an enormous host and bring it down.

Neat huh? But not good if you are the victim.

However this remarkable discovery by Bassler has two important consequences, both with enormous medical implications.

A whole new type of antibiotics can be looked for, which will effectively block the quorum sensing molecules (like jamming the enemy radar).

Health can be built, helping to block out bad bacteria, by supporting and provoking the chemical sensing of the good, friendly bacteria that support us!

Watch out, this is the way it's going to go.

Meantime, we have to worry about protecting ourselves.

What about viruses?

Viruses, are dangerous and can cause many infectious diseases, some of which can be fatal to humans. Smallpox, for example. However, viruses are not the same as bacteria. While a bacterium is a single celled organism, a virus is not even a single cell; technically it's the equivalent of part of a nucleus—just a package of DNA, wrapped up in a protein envelope.

The virus cannot live and cannot reproduce, unless it breaks into a cell and hijacks the cell's reproductive mechanism. It does this by taking over the DNA of the cell and forcing the cell to replicate its own viral DNA. This results in making lots of new viruses, but the cell will usually die in this process, releasing the new viruses to go and infect more cells. So the disease spreads.

The trouble is, viruses are not killed by antibiotics so, although they may be very dangerous, they don't come under the material covered by this report. Only a few anti-viral substances are available, and none which are fully safe. But that's a different story.

What about parasites?

Parasites are different again. They may cause disease and can be either single celled or multicellular animals. A worm, for example is multi-celled; as well as mechanisms for digestion, it has muscular fibers for movement.

Segmented worms, like tapeworms, are certainly multicellular, but each segment is more or less identical to the segment above and segment below. So parasites of this type work a bit like a duplicating or photocopying machine, breaking off new pieces of identical infected tissue and eggs. It's more like a colony than an animal, really.

But we also have single cell parasites such as Giardia lamblia and malaria.

Yes, malaria is a parasitic disease; the killer organism of the species Falciparum invades the blood and reproduces itself destroying blood cells in the process. The patient will sometimes die of too much blood loss as much as the severe fever which can ensue.

Note that the infamous mosquito is only the spreader of the malaria parasite. It does not otherwise cause malaria and you may be bitten by a mosquito and not get malaria. Conversely, you cannot get malaria unless you are bitten by an infected mosquito. The mosquito is an essential intermediate we call a "vector".

There are many treatments for parasites depending on the nature of the organism concerned. None of these fall within the definition of antibiotic, and so will not be considered in this report.

Where there is a clear vector, such as in the case of malaria, wiping out the vector is an obvious way to block transmission of the disease. However trying to eliminate mosquitoes has met with only very limited success. That doesn't seem to be the way to go.

Historic antibacterials

Many cures for infectious diseases existed prior to the beginning of the twentieth century which were based on medicinal folklore. That didn't mean they did not work; just that doctors weren't interested in them!

Cures for infection in ancient Chinese medicine, using plants with antibiotic-like properties, began to be described over 2,500 years ago. Many other ancient cultures, including the ancient Egyptians, ancient Greeks and medieval Arabs already used molds and plants to treat infections.

Cinchona bark (quinine) was a widely effective treatment of malaria in the 17th century, the disease caused by protozoan parasites of the genus Plasmodium.

According to legend, the first European ever to be cured from malaria fever was the wife of the Spanish Viceroy, the countess of Chinchon (hence the name).

The court physician was summoned and urged to save the countess from the waves of fever and chill that were threatening her life, but every effort failed to relieve her. At last the physician administered some medicine which he had obtained from the local Indians, who had been using it for similar syndromes. The countess survived the malarial attack and reportedly brought the cinchona bark back with her when she returned to Europe in the 1640s.

The birth of homeopathy (see section #41) was based on quinine testing. The founder of homeopathy, Dr. Samuel Hahnemann, when translating the Cullen's Materia medica, noticed that Dr. Cullen wrote that quinine cures malaria and can also produce malaria. Dr. Hahnemann took daily a large non-homeopathic dose of quinine bark. After two weeks, he said he felt malaria-like symptoms. This idea of "like cures like" was the starting point of his writings on "Homeopathy".

The Love Triangle

Gonorrhea, together with syphilis and HIV, make a "love triangle" of the most famous sexually transmitted diseases. Indeed, gonorrhea, caused by the Neisseria gonorrhoeae bacterium, affects 62 million people, aged mainly 15 to 29, and represents the world's second most widespread STDs after the infection with Chlamydia trachomatis (930,000 cases of Chlamydial infection and 360,000 of gonorrhea were assessed in the United States in 2004).

But the power of gonorrhea is what really has shocked the scientists (as revealed in a new research published in PLoS Biology): relative to its weight, the Neisseria bacterium is the strongest organism on Earth: it can pull up to 100,000 times its body weight (could you drag 7,000 tons?).

Many bacteria move around using up to 10 contractile filaments named pili. The pili can be 10 times longer than the bacterium itself. Neisseria bacteria employ pili, but no one has seen before that these bacteria can join the force of their pili for achieving long, strong pulls.

The team led by Michael Sheetz at Columbia University in New York

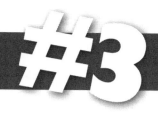

#3 Staphylococcus and Co.

Now let's get back to bacterial disease and the problems we face trying to eliminate them.

I want to emphasize that Staphylococcus infections have been with humankind since forever. Most infections affect the skin and are mild. S. aureus was first identified in Aberdeen, Scotland, in 1880 by the surgeon Sir Alexander Ogston in pus from surgical abscesses [Classics In Infectious Diseases. "On Abscesses". Alexander Ogston (1844-1929)].

The name Staphylococcus aureus (abbreviated to S. aureus or Staph aureus in medical literature), literally means the "golden cluster seed" or "seed gold" . It is named on account of its golden appearance when it grows in colonies. You have probably seen the color too, in the golden-yellow crusts that form on the face, around the mouth, called impetigo.

About 20% of the population are long-term carriers of S. aureus. It can cause a range of illnesses from minor skin infections, such as pimples, impetigo, boils, cellulitis, folliculitis, carbuncles and abscesses, to life-threatening diseases such as pneumonia, meningitis, osteomyelitis, endocarditis, Toxic shock syndrome (TSS), and septicemia.

The new antibiotic resistant MRSA monster has been created by doctors, not by Nature. For years it has been the feared hospital bug that no-one talks about, because it's something given to you by doctors and nurses when you enter their environment. A survey earlier this year suggested that MRSA infections, including noninvasive mild forms, affect as many as 5 percent of hospital patients. Nobody wants suing; hence the secrecy.

Nobody likes to be a bringer of bad news but it is clearly going to get worse. More deaths. Hospitals are becoming a horribly unsafe place to be.

Beware of the hospitals!

Hospitals are just about the most UN-healthy places a person can find themselves. The very people who are looking after you, may be giving you a very unpleasant disease. One in every 20 healthcare workers carries methicillin-resistant Staphylococcus aureus (MRSA), researchers in Switzerland said.

But the vast majority is without symptoms and only 5% have full-blown clinical infections, according to Stephan Harbarth, M.D., of the University Hospitals of Geneva, and Werner Albrich, M.D., of University Hospital Bern.

One implication is that screening efforts aimed at symptomatic infections are likely to miss a large proportion of colonized healthcare workers who might transmit the bacteria, according to a review in the May 2008 issue of Lancet Infectious Diseases.

Instead, the study authors said, "aggressive screening and eradication policies" should be used in an outbreak and in situations where MRSA has not reached highly endemic levels. The researchers looked at 127 studies published from January 1980 through March 2006, to see how likely healthcare workers are to be infected or colonized by MRSA and to assess their role in MRSA transmission.

On the basis of the published evidence, the study said, healthcare workers are usually vectors, rather than the main sources of MRSA transmission, implying that "good hand hygiene practices remain essential to control the spread of MRSA."

Among 33,318 workers screened in the studies, 4.6% on average were carrying MRSA, the researchers found -- usually in the nose, although other sites were found. Most (94.9%) had no symptoms.

Risk factors included chronic skin diseases, poor hygiene practices, and having worked in countries with endemic MRSA.

Research revealed 18 studies with proven, and 26 studies with likely, transmission to patients from healthcare workers who were not clinically infected with MRSA.

"Staphylococcal dispersal is mainly dependent on whether the person is a nasal carrier," researchers said, so that "screening of infected healthcare workers only will likely miss a large number of asymptomatic personnel capable of transmitting MRSA to patients."

So beware!

Source reference: Albrich WC, Harbarth S "Health-care workers: Source, vector, or victim of MRSA?" Lancet Infect Dis 2008; 8: 289-301.

Pets Can Give You MRSA Too

Pet owners are blithely unaware that life-threatening pathogens can be picked up from their beloved pooch or pussycat.

According to Dr. Richard Oehler, of the University of South Florida College of Medicine in Tampa, and colleagues writing in the July 2009 issue of The Lancet Infectious Diseases.

Dog and cat bites account for about 1% of emergency department visits each year in the United States and Europe. Severe infections occur in about 20% of all cases and are caused by bacteria from the animal's mouth, plus possibly other bacteria from the human patient's skin.

About one in every 10 dogs or cats carries S. aureus. About a third (35%) of those were found to carry the MRSA strain, according to a study done at the University of Pennsylvania Veterinary School.

Of course infections travel both ways. More human cases of community-acquired MRSA leads to more MRSA colonization in domestic animals.

In fact, the study found that in some cases, pets may be picking the pathogen up from humans. "A growing body of clinical evidence has documented MRSA colonization in domestic animals, often implying direct acquisition of S. aureus infection from their human owners," the team noted. MRSA-related skin infections in pets can then easily spread back to humans, so your pet may pose considerable danger.

Sepsis, a potentially fatal bloodstream infection, can be a complication following bite wounds from a pet infected with MRSA or other types of bacteria.

Animals bites are a major cause of injury in the USA and Europe each year, particularly in children. Bites to the hands, forearms, neck and head are usually the worst.

Treatment of MRSA infections in pets is similar to that used in humans and for the most part, the danger to pet owners -- even those most vulnerable to MRSA -- remains low.

SOURCE: The Lancet Infectious Diseases, news release, June 21, 2009 The worry now is that MRSA has spread beyond hospitals into the community. It's fancy name is CA-MRSA (community-associated methicillin-resistant staphylococcus aureus). In recent years, the resistant germ has been spreading through prisons, gyms and school locker rooms, mostly in poor urban neighborhoods.

An especially dangerous form is brought about by inhalation; the bacteria goes straight to the lungs, produces a sudden and violent pneumonia and the victim can die WITHIN HOURS, coughing up frothy blood and unable to breathe.

This is why I likened it to the Black Death (Bubonic Plague or just "The Plague"). The so-called respiratory form of Plague in olden times was also very sudden; it often killed the same day as it was inhaled. Remember the kid's nursery rhyme "Tissue, aTissue, We all Fall down" (dead)? That was said to commemorate respiratory Bubonic plague.

Suddenly, queues and public gatherings are potentially dangerous places. You are just as likely to catch this modern killer in a queue at the supermarket, from some young all-American sports youth or cheerleader, as you are from a foreigner, so please do not start or join any aversion campaign against "dirty immigrants". It's ignorant and could cost YOU your life by having you focus on the wrong thing.

Community Active MRSA

The worry now is that MRSA has spread beyond hospitals into the community. It's fancy name is CA-MRSA (community-associated methicillin-resistant staphylococcus aureus). In recent years, the resistant germ has been spreading through prisons, gyms and school locker rooms, mostly in poor urban neighborhoods.

An especially dangerous form is brought about by inhalation; the bacteria goes straight to the lungs, produces a sudden and violent pneumonia and the victim can die WITHIN HOURS, coughing up frothy blood and unable to breathe.

This is why I likened it to the Black Death (Bubonic Plague or just "The Plague"). The so-called respiratory form of Plague in olden times was also very sudden; it often killed the same day as it was inhaled. Remember the kid's nursery rhyme "Tissue, aTissue, We all Fall down" (dead)? That was said to commemorate respiratory Bubonic plague.

Suddenly, queues and public gatherings are potentially dangerous places. You are just as likely to catch this modern killer in a queue at the supermarket, from some young all-American sports youth or cheerleader, as you are from a foreigner, so please do not start or join any aversion campaign against "dirty immigrants". It's ignorant and could cost YOU your life by having you focus on the wrong thing.

#4 The Danger Is Increasing

Exactly as I predicted in the first edition of this book, things are falling apart rapidly. We are just a few years from total meltdown.

In 2009 a new strain of MRSA arose which is more deadly than anything we have seen previously. According to a report (November 1st 2009) this new strain of MRSA is five times more lethal than what has gone before. The mortality is 50%, compared to 11% for the "normal" MRSA [Henry Ford Hospital study presented at the 47th annual meeting of the Infectious Diseases Society of America Oct. 29-Nov.1 in Philadelphia].

Why aren't the newspapers and TV programs screaming about this?

Bear in mind, the problem here is not just MRSA. Now we have Vancomycin resistant enterococcus (VRE). That's much more to be feared: if it reaches the septicemia stage it is 100% fatal. Nothing can stop it (Vancomycin is known as the "last defence" antibiotic).

Our old killer enemy TB has now morphed into a new strain which is resistant to ALL KNOWN ANTIBIOTIC DRUGS.

Also we now have PRSP (penicillin-resistant Streptococcus pneumoniae). It is reported that out of 100,000 hospitalizations for pneumonia, 40% are now due to this organism.

Then there is GISA. Never heard of that one?

In December 2002 the microbiology department at Monklands Hospital, Scotland isolated only the third Glycopeptide Intermediate Staph Aureus (GISA) in the United Kingdom.

The press were involved due to the rarity of this organism and the fact that this infection had a fatal outcome for the patient (the first fatal case in the UK). After a press conference, Dr Alistair Leanord, consultant microbiologist, invited TV crews into the microbiology department to film biomedical scientist staff using the Vitek Autoanalyser, which was used to initially detect the GISA organism.

The problem is, GISA is not susceptible to vancomycin or teicoplanin. Vancomycin and teicoplanin are considered the last line of defence against

MRSA. However, fortunately, all GISA isolates to date have been susceptible to other antimicrobial drugs that have been effective in treating cases.

But what happens when that lucky state of affairs runs out?

C. difficile and membranous ulcerative colitis

You may have heard of C. difficile (or C. dif and various other appelations). Its real name is Clostridium difficile and that says it all. Most of the Clostridia species are nasty and cause diseases like botulism and gas gangrene. Diff causes membranous ulcerative colitis, a severe and often fatal bowel inflammation.

Dif comes about from overuse and abuse of antibiotics. It's just another example of where good turns bad; the wonders of antibiotics become a deadly liability.

In recent years, C. difficile infections have become more frequent, more severe and more difficult to treat. The European Center for Disease Prevention and Control recommend that fluoroquinolones and the antibiotic clindamycin be avoided in clinical practice due to their high association with subsequent Clostridium difficile infections.

The emergence of a new, highly toxic strain of C. difficile, resistant to fluoroquinolone antibiotics, such as ciprofloxacin (Cipro) and levofloxacin (Levaquin), said to be causing geographically dispersed outbreaks in North America was reported in 2005. The Centers for Disease Control in Atlanta has also warned of the emergence of an epidemic strain with increased virulence, antibiotic resistance, or both [McDonald L (2005). "Clostridium difficile: responding to a new threat from an old enemy" (PDF). Infect Control Hosp Epidemiol 26 (8): 672–5. doi:10.1086/502600. PMID 16156321].

When severe, symptoms include watery diarrhea 10 to 15 times a day, abdominal cramping and pain, fever, blood or pus in the stool, nausea, dehydration and loss of weight.

Some people may be symptom free carriers (as with amebic dysentry).

Treatment is difficult, wouldn't you know!

Antidiarrheals are strictly contraindicated because a life-threatening dilation of the bowel called toxic megacolon may result.

Different antibiotics may be called for. Treatment with oral vancomycin or parenteral metronidazole usually will result in abatement of symptoms within 3 to 5 days.

This is certainly one puppy that isn't going to yield to yoghourt and roughage!

But unless the patient needs hospitalizing for support, chlorine dioxide therapy (section #18) should be tried; hydrogen peroxide (section #19); or colloidal silver (section #21).

Probiotics are essential. The orthodox treatment of choice is rapidly becoming a human faecal transplant (see section 40b).

A SCENAR (section #44) and homeopathics (section #41), would bring in useful energetic support. Try Cantharis, Colchicum, Colocynthis, Arg.Nit., Brom., Lach.

Aloe vera is the best herb to try (section #35).

#5 The Golden Age Is Over!

In an article which appeared in Medscape, 2/3/2010, Dr Paul Auwaerter, MD, MBA, Clinical Director, Division of Infectious Diseases at Johns Hopkins University School of Medicine, was quoted as saying that, "The patients are sicker than ever before, so we are using antibiotics more intensively, and the bacteria are changing in response. At the same time we have really lost ground in incentive mechanisms for creation and production of new antimicrobial compounds."

Emerging Antibiotics: Will We Have What We Need? Laura A. Stokowski, RN, MS

Unfortunately, the general public are still not getting this problem of antibiotic resistance or the absence of effective new antibiotics. People generally have faith or have been lulled into believing that medical scientists can develop effective new antibiotics whenever needed because they have always done so in the past.

By the time most people wake up to the realities of the situation, it will be too late. Antibiotic-resistant infections are becoming the next great equalizer, and this is not just a problem for the elderly or the immune-suppressed. Friends and family, rich and poor alike, will succumb to infections that should be curable but aren't, and everyone will be looking around for someone to blame.

The many factors that have contributed to the current crisis have already been debated, but these sobering facts remain:

- More US patients die of MRSA infections than HIV/AIDS and tuberculosis combined.

- Only 2 new antibiotics -- doripenem and telavancin -- have been approved in the past 3 years.

- We have no drugs to treat infections with some strains of multi-drug-resistant gram-negative bacilli, like Pseudomonas aeruginosa and Actinobacter baumannii.

We may finally have arrived at the era of the untreatable bacterial infection.

Livermore DM. Has the era of untreatable infections arrived? J Antimicrob Chemother. 2009;64(Suppl 1):29-36.

Mechanisms are varied

Resistance can be either inherent -- as exemplified by the inability of vancomycin to penetrate the cell wall of gram-negative bacteria -- or acquired. Acquired resistance is a change in the bacterium's genetic composition that permits clinical resistance to drugs that were once active against it. Acquired resistance can reduce the effectiveness of an antibiotic or render the antibiotic completely ineffective against the bacterium.

Bacteria can also become resistant to other classes of antibiotics (cross-resistance) or transfer their resistance genes to other microbes and species (co-resistance). The strategies used by bacteria to resist the actions of antibiotics include:

- Reduced outer membrane permeability;

- Reduced cytoplasmic membrane transport;

- Increased efflux/decreased influx of antibiotic;

- Neutralization of antibiotic by enzymes;

- Target modification; and

- Target elimination

SOURCE: Chen LF, Chopra T, Kaye KS. Pathogens resistant to antibacterial agents. Infect Dis Clin N Am. 2009;23:817-845

Escape Pathogens
(usually labeled ESKAPE)

These are pathogens of highest concern; the most serious, life-threatening infections as classified by the Infectious Diseases Society of America (IDSA), so-called because they effectively escape the effects of antibacterial drugs.

These include:

- E Enterococcus faecium Third most common cause of health-care associated blood stream infections. Increasing resistance to vancomycin.

- S Staphylococcus aureus (MRSA) Emerging resistance to current drugs and significant

- drug toxicities. Lack of oral agents for step-down therapy

- K Klebsiella

- Escherichia coli

- K pneumoniae Extended beta-lactamase producing organisms increasing in frequency and severity; associated with increasing mortality. K pneumoniae carbapenemases causing severe infections in LTCF. Few active agents; nothing in development

- A Acinetobacter baumannii Increasing worldwide, recent surge reported in hospitals. Very high mortality. Carbapenem-resistant.

- P Pseudomonas aeruginosa Increasing P. aeruginosa infections in US and worldwide. Resistant to carbapenems, quinolones, aminoglycosides

- E Enterobacter species MDR HCA infections increasing; resistance via ESBLs, carbapenemases, and cephalosporinases

(**key:** HCA = healthcare associated; BSI = bloodstream infection; MRSA = methicillin resistant S aureus; ESBL = extended-spectrum beta-lactamase; LTCF = long-term care facility; MDR = multiple drug-resistant)

No New Antiobiotics On The Way

The trouble is, according to Brad Spellberg, MD, Associate Professor of Medicine, Geffen School of Medicine at UCLA, "The economic and regulatory climates have changed so that the drug companies aren't making new antibiotics. We've been talking about antibiotic stewardship since the 1950s. It used to be 'new bug, new drug,' but not anymore. We are already seeing infections resistant to all of the antibiotics that we have now, and the number will increase at a geometric rate over the next 5 years."

It's not that there aren't any antibiotics in development. There are, but they won't solve our real problems. The antibiotics aimed at gram-negative infections that are currently in development have mechanisms of action similar to the drugs we already have available. Ceftobiprole and ceftaroline, for example, have both completed phase 3 trials, but they are essentially the same as cefepime, a drug already on the market. A gram-negative organism resistant to cefepime, then, will also be resistant to both ceftobiprole and ceftaroline. So, explains Dr. Spellberg, the real problem is that there are no gram-negative antibiotics in the pipeline that will work against bacteria already resistant to the drugs we have. The number of drugs that have made it through the developmental process and received FDA approval has plummeted in recent years. From 1983 through 2007, systemic antibacterial approvals declined by 75%. *[Boucher HW, Talbot GH, Bradley JS, et al. Bad bugs, no drugs, no ESKAPE! An update from the Infectious Diseases Society of America. Clin Infect Dis. 2009;48:1-12. Abstract].*

What the Rest of Us Can Do

Dr. Paul Auwaerter has 2 suggestions: First, education and awareness of this issue must increase among the medical community. Second, political, and scientific forces must work together to recognize the scope of the problem and develop solutions. "We learned a lesson from the H1N1 pandemic: the importance of being prepared. Right now, we are not close to being adequately prepared."

We need to realize that it isn't just our patients who are at risk, it's all of us. But nothing will change if we sit back and think this problem is too big, too complex, that it's someone else's problem, or that there is nothing we can do. There is something we must do, according to Dr. Spellberg. "Only when constituents start putting pressure on elected officials will things change."

"We need [physicians' and nurses'] voices because right now the FDA is dominated by statisticians and the clinicians are being shouted down. We have lost our voices. They are making drug approval decisions based on statistical results and have lost all sight of clinical reality."

Dr. Spellberg recommends writing letters to the editors of professional journals or other media, expressing concern -- and yes, outrage -- about the current situation. People can also inform regulatory officials and politicians that the current approach to approving drugs is unacceptable; that physicians are being excluded from these conversations, and that statisticians should not have the sole voice. Demand that the FDA stop insisting on perfection and demand that clinicians have a say in the approval process. DO YOUR PART: read this important information manual and raise your voice. Only by wide public action will anything change. The dangers are real; they are here NOW and are not (ever) going to go away. So take immediate action.

The Bottom Line

"As the Medscape article concluded: We are literally inches away from a crisis in public health that will severely hamper our ability to transplant organs, replace hips, provide cancer chemotherapy, perform dialysis, or keep premature babies alive. Then, it will only be a matter of time before otherwise healthy individuals will die because they contracted infections after routine surgery or were infected by pathogens that are common in the community but for which we no longer have a cure." Death is stalking everybody. Get wise; get educated and take effective action.

My Advice

I can tell you that the usual trite advice: using chlorox or Lysol and washing your hands is a waste of time against the pneumonic form. Shocked? You shouldn't be. Count on "official" recommendations to be stupid, inadequate and/or worthless.

They don't even listen to their own science.

The question remains: if there is a pandemic of this organism, what should you do? Please note that my answers amount to good health advice for the present, when and while you remain fit and well. This is not just "disaster talk". Any good health measure is a good protection measure in the event of an epidemic or pandemic. Those who survive will do so because they have strong physiology and a vibrant immune system.

You can forget the idea that the doctor will come along and help you. Even if the medical profession knew how to deal with such a problem (which it doesn't), there would simply not be enough doctors to go around. You will be on your own.

But don't panic. Contact does not mean inevitably going down with the disease. Millions did not die in the Plague years. Those who worked the carts to carry off the dead bodies generally survived: it was NOT a suicide job! Doctors don't all fall over with the diseases they treat, even though they are in intimate contact with infected patients.

What is important is to build good health; overall health.

In addition, you need to know some very handy treatments that will kill pathogens as effectively as prescription drugs. You have not been told about these—and you are not likely to be, with the establishment taking its orders from the trans-national pharmaceutical cartels (trans-national really translates as they don't obey any country's laws).

The fact is these humble remedies I shall list are mostly cheap and there is not much profit in them. Not enough for greedy directors and stockholders of the drug companies.

This eReport will introduce you to DOZENS of modalities for treating and eliminating infectious bacterial pathogens. Many of the treatments, incidentally, will also work against viruses AND parasites, which is more than can be said for antibiotics.

But first, we have some study to do! As the sun begins to set on the magic of antibiotics and the (apparent) safety they brought, you need to learn what we are up against for the future.

This eReport will introduce you to DOZENS of modalities for treating and eliminating infectious bacterial pathogens. Many of the treatments, incidentally, will also work against viruses AND parasites, which is more than can be said for antibiotics.

But first, we have some study to do! As the sun begins to set on the magic of antibiotics and the (apparent) safety they brought, you need to learn what we are up against for the future.

Part 1

Understanding The Enemy

#6 Our fight with bacteria

There are approximately ten times as many bacterial cells as human cells in the human body, with large numbers of bacteria on the skin and in the digestive tract. The vast majority of the bacteria in the body are rendered harmless by the protective effects of the immune system, and a few are beneficial.

However, a few species of bacteria are pathogenic and cause infectious diseases, including cholera, syphilis, anthrax, leprosy and bubonic plague. The most common fatal bacterial diseases are respiratory infections, with tuberculosis alone killing about 2 million people a year, mostly in sub-Saharan Africa.

For a time we got ahead in the war against infectious diseases. Better nutrition and public hygiene have been the main reason for the improvements. Vaccinations seem to be mainly a waste of time and have made no real impact on the gradual disappearance of infectious diseases.

There is no question that antibiotics, too, made a huge impact in this war. For a time we had better weapons and ammunition than the enemy; it was only natural we would win. But even as antibiotics triumphed, within just a few years of their birth, resistant germs began to appear.

The implications of this were being discussed even in my time as a med. student in the 1960s. But nobody really paid much attention. The relentless advertizing and heavy pushes of the antibiotic manufacturers, coupled with the natural human tendency to laziness on the part of doctors, meant that the drug industry went on making huge profits. And all the while, the time bomb was ticking.

Back then we were just too naïve to understand or care about the possible long-term consequences of excessive prescriptions. Today, with 20/20 hindsight, we can say the path to where we are has been marked by reckless folly and greed.

We have arrived at a place where the short-comings of drug-based medicine are all too plain.

Antibiotics are gradually ceasing to work; most drugs have little real benefit and lots of side effects; the costs of prescriptions has risen to the point where drugs are now a huge proportion of the gross national product and deaths due to medicines has soared to the point where, in the US alone, iatrogenic deaths—deaths caused by doctors—are now over 100,000 per year.

That's more citizens than were killed by the entire 10 years of the Vietnam war!

And when I say drug deaths, I mean where the CORRECT drug, was CORRECTLY PRESCRIBED. Mistakes and blunders account for a further 7,000 deaths per year. And that's from a study carried out by a professor of medicine at Johns Hopkins School of Hygiene and Public Health, not "statistics" from left wing agitators or Ralph Nader.

[By the way, since it is germaine to the topic in question, you can throw in another 80,000 deaths a year from infections acquired in hospital and despite the very best of antibiotic therapy].

Not a pretty picture.

But the other way our world has been SERIOUSLY DAMAGED is by the obsession with finding the pharmaceutical "holy grail" is that basic medicine and health care has been lost.

Doctors don't even consider hygiene these days. They just fall back on antibiotics.

A study published in the Annals of Internal Medicine (2004), brought to light the fact that doctors, even surgeons, who thought they were not being watched, didn't bother to wash their hands much. They were caught on a hidden video camera.

This is despite the proof from Dr. Ignaz Semmelweiss, going back over a century, that surgeons washing their hands before an operation saved the lives of countless women in childbed (puerperal sepsis or "childbed fever" had over 50- 100% mortality and it was mainly caused by poor hygiene technique).

In this study, under an infection control expert with the University of Geneva Hospitals, researchers sought to better understand doctors' attitudes. They secretly tracked 163 doctors to monitor their hand washing during the day. Each doctor also completed a survey about their attitudes on hand hygiene.

They observed just 57% of doctors washing their hands between patients. Internists and medical students were the most diligent about washing their hands. Surgeons and anesthesiologists washed their hands least often.

On days when doctors had a busy workload, they were less likely to wash, the report shows. If they thought they were being watched, they were more likely to wash.

If doctors carried hand-wipe packets with them, or if hand-rub solutions were at the patient's bedside, they were more likely to use them. These solutions don't require water and a sink.

In fact, an expert infection-control panel recently issued a national recommendation promoting the use of these hand-rub solutions for disinfecting hands that are not grossly soiled, writes Robert A. Weinstein, MD, with Chicago's Cook County Hospital, in an accompanying editorial.

It's "excellent advice," he writes. Doctors "must use these products as a matter of ritual on entering and leaving every patient's room." Also, doctors must act as role models for medical students to ensure that each generation of doctors follows good hand hygiene -- and infection control -- practices.

It's not just hygiene

It's worse. Doctors no longer think of healthy nutrition. Yet that's the whole reason we beat TB. This disease was nearly gone before the first antibiotics arrived in the 1950s. TB is a disease of under-nutrition. Good food is the cure, not drugs and certainly not the vaccine (BCG).

Rest, calm, good food and love are the main ingredients of any good medical practice. Yet these are ignored, in the stupid belief they are unimportant and that drugs are the "real" medicine. Hell, people recovered all over the place before these drugs were ever invented.

There are some truths that will never go away, no matter what scientific advances may come about. Doctors who lose sight of these healing elements are a danger to the community.

Finally, as you know, countless safe and effective remedies from popular culture were summarily dropped as if they had no place in modern medicine. Herbs and other remedies have been around for centuries: they are not here because people are gullible and believe in folk myth and snake oil—but because these herbs really do work!

Homeopathy too has proven itself time and again. Now it is virtually banned and doctors who practice it treated as outlaws.

The result?

We are going downhill rapidly to a dangerous new time, when drugs may not be able to dig us out of the mess caused by doctor folly. I am concerned.

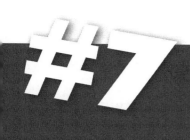

#7 Killing Bacteria Has A Downside

Even killing pathogens can wreak havoc. Consider this cautionary tale: it shows we have a lot more to learn.

When scientists discovered that a bacterium Helicobacter pylori, not stress, caused most stomach ulcers, two researchers were awarded a 2005 Nobel Prize and medical practice changed significantly. Now antibiotics are used to treat ulcers. It is satisfying to note that ulcers and even stomach cancers have declined dramatically in numbers.

However microbiologist Martin Blaser and his colleagues at New York University began to document an odd medical trend. As Helicobacter pylori, virtually disappeared among children, cases of asthma tripled. So did rates of hay fever and allergies, such as eczema.

After analyzing health records of 7,412 people collected by the National Center for Health Statistics, Dr. Blaser and NYU epidemiologist Yu Chen reported this summer (2009) in the Journal of Infectious Diseases that children between three and 13 years old who tested positive for H. pylori bacteria were 59% less likely to have asthma. They also were 40% to 60% less likely to have hay fever or rashes.

Among adults, gastro-esophageal reflux disease (GERD) became more common, as did some forms of esophageal cancer.

Dr. Blaser soon reasoned that eliminating the harm these bacteria cause is at the expense of the protection they provide us. He may be right. The jury is still out.

One thing is for sure: we are landlords to an immense host of bacteria and most of these species, and what effects they may have, are still unknown to science. But we must now suspect that they interact with us in diverse ways and can influence obesity, heart disease and cancer, as well as many other conditions.

As many as 500 species of bacteria may inhabit our guts, like H.pylori. Maybe 500 or so other species make themselves at home in our mouth, where each tooth has its own unique bacterial colony. No one knows how many species we contain in all. This past August, researchers at Kings

College London identified yet another new species of oral bacteria between the tongue and cheek.

We are the equivalent of an Amazonian rain forest, where they discover new species every week!

Until recently, half of humanity carried Herlicobacter pylori stomach bacteria, according to a 2002 study in the New England Journal of Medicine. Indeed, we appear to have evolved together. Among those born in the U.S. under the age of 25 or so, only 5% or so still carry Helicobacter, largely due to the indiscriminate use of antibiotics.

The connection to allergies is just one of the pressing public health puzzles posed by our complex relationship with the trillions of microbes that call us home. "Recent studies have shown that changes in bacteria can be correlated with some pretty serious diseases," says Jane Peterson, head of the National Human Genome Research Institute's comparative sequencing program.

Childhood diabetes also is on the rise in developed countries, for instance. Last week, University of Chicago immunologist Alexander Chervonsky and his collaborators at Yale University reported that doses of beneficial stomach bacteria can stop the development of Type 1 diabetes in lab mice.

Common stomach bacteria also can stop the development of Type 1 diabetes in lab mice, researchers have reported. The researchers believe their findings could one day be used to develop bacteria-based treatments for patients.

Other bacteria are just as crucial to our well-being, feeding us the calories from food we can't digest on our own, bolstering our immune systems, tending our skin and dosing us with vitamins, such as B6 and B12, which we are unable to synthesize unaided.

So indiscriminate use of antibiotics may carry a whole host of complications that cannot be foreseen. For sure, we will disturb the natural balance and for that we have a term: dysbiosis. It is particularly important in the gut, where dysbiosis can lead to multiple health problems, including food allergies and overgrowth of less friendly yeasts and bacteria.

Metagenomics May Give Us The Edge

Now scientists are trying to sequence bacterial genes (like plotting the human genome). No-one knows what will emerge from an investigation like this. But it's being taken very seriously. In 2008 the National Institutes of Health launched a 5-year, $125 million Human Micro-biome Project to analyze hundreds of microbial species that make your body their home.

Making the project possible is a new gene-mapping technique called metagenomics.

To start, researchers at the Baylor College of Medicine in Houston, the Washington University School of Medicine in St. Louis, the Broad Institute in Cambridge, Mass., and the J. Craig Venter Institute in Rockville, Md., have been sequencing the genomes of 200 microbe species isolated from 250 healthy volunteers. They are sampling bacteria from the skin, gut, vagina, mouth and nose, then attempting to identify them by cataloging variations in a single gene sequence that all bacteria share.

Working with similar metagenomics projects in Europe, Japan, China and Canada, they hope to assemble a reference collection of genomic information covering 1,000 microbial species that infest us. If all goes as planned, they may soon find themselves trying to analyze 200,000 genes, compared to a feeble 20,000 for the human genome.

These data sets are so huge, and we don't have the tools yet to analyze them. But the diversity is more than anyone expected. Dr. Segre, who specializes in the study of the skin, found one set of microbial communities thriving in the bend of the typical elbow and an entirely different set of colonies on the average forearm.

In all, she identified 113 different kinds of bacteria living in concentrations of about 10,000 per square centimeter on the surface and, just beneath the skin, in densities of one million microbes per square centimeter, she reported last May.

In a real sense, the history of all these many microbes is the history of humanity itself. "We are living beings that co-evolved with micro-organisms," Dr. Segre says. Evidence suggests that strains of helicobacter bacteria evolved along with humankind from its beginnings in primitive organisms a billion years ago. Every mammalian species appears to have its own unique variety of these microbes. Human-strain Helicobacter pylori accompanied our anatomically modern ancestors on their great walk out of Africa about 58,000 years ago. Molecular epidemiologists at the Max Planck Institute for

Infection Biology in Berlin have so far identified 370 strains of the bacteria that seemed to reflect the migrations and settlements of their human hosts.

It is vital that we understand bacteria better, like this, rather than just thinking in crude terms of antiseptics and antibiotic drugs.

#8 The rise of the superbugs

The greatest old-time "superbug" was the one that brought the ravages of the "Black Death". That's the dread plague that swept the world in waves, over the 13th – 17th century. At its peak, it wiped out one third of the known population of the world. Imagine that today. Two billion people; where would we put all those bodies? We'd need machinery to dig graves fast enough. Decayed people would ooze into our water table.

However today, I don't think we would lose such a big proportion of folks, because of antibiotics. But what would happen if antibiotics began to fail us, as they are beginning to do? It's hard for younger people born today to imagine what such a world would be like.

You'd have to be over 70 years to remember back to a time like that. I'm in my sixties and, as a baby boomer, was born right at the start of the penicillin era.

But there were still cases walking the streets that you just wouldn't see today. Like the kid in our village who had his right arm amputated at the shoulder. I was puzzled and upset by his deformity. Then the adults explained he'd nicked his finger on a tin can, got gangrene and had to lose his arm to save his life.

Later in life, while I was at med school, there were still cases showing the era of the "old medicine". Congenital syphilis, for example. It shows with a collapsed nose bridge and punched out holes, like extra nostrils , sucking air right through the sides. You could see that on a public 'bus quite regularly (though of course the syphilis had eventually been eradicated in that person's body, by the judicious use of antibiotics).

The late stages of syphilis were in evidence right up to the 1970s. General paresis of the insane (GPI, so-called) was the outrageous one, almost funny, characterized by megalomania. One patient when I was at medical school declared he was God, escaped the hospital and tried to buy a building for a million (he had no money), swept up to a minor radio celebrity and proposed to her and was finally picked up by the police "shooting the rapids" in a sewage facility.

It has been speculated that Nietsche, a megalomaniac philosopher if ever there was one, suffered with GPI. Following a psychotic breakdown in 1889, at the age of 44 years, he was admitted to the Basel mental asylum and on

41

18 January 1889 was transferred to the Jena mental asylum. He remained in demented darkness until his death on 25 August 1900. In Basel, a diagnosis of general paralysis of the insane (GPI; tertiary cerebral syphilis) was made.

This diagnosis was confirmed in Jena and is still widely accepted.

But easier to see, walking down the street, was Tabes dorsalis. This wretched condition is characterized by a stamping gait, due to loss of leg co-ordination. But the worst aspect, from the patient's point of view, are the stabbing agonizing pains in the back and down the leg. Poor Delius, the composer, had this.

Ironically, normal nerve signals didn't get through. The patient would smash up their own knee joints, etc. because the protective mechanisms were not in place. It's a moral lesson in the fact that pain is really there to protect us from harm, not make us miserable.

Why am I wasting my time on this despicable disease, some may ask? Because syphilis was one of the most feared of all diseases for centuries and kept young men and women in terror of the act of union. It cast its dark shadow over saints and sinners alike and many a creative genius was snuffed out by its chill wind.

Trust me, you would not want this monster to break loose again. Yet antibiotic-resistant syphilis has been with us for decades, certainly since the Vietnam war. GIs on furlough, young tarts who want to make cash giving them sex and bad prescribing by military MDs made it almost inevitable.

All those romantic Victorian novels

Who hasn't read Dickens and Jane Austen and all those great old-time stories? Often one of the characters takes ill and dies, almost immediately. You wonder why?

The dreaded diseases were TB (a very slow death, due to consumption) and lobar pneumonia. The latter was once nicknamed "Captain Of The White Horsemen Of Death", due to its terrifying swiftness. A person would get wet on Friday and take a chill, develop a fever on Saturday and be dead by bedtime on Sunday. There was no treatment as such, all the doctor and family could do was wait for the "crisis".

This is the moment you have seen often in movies and on TV; the patient's fever rages higher and higher and they rave in delirium. The loving wife sits there helplessly mopping the sweat from the patient's brow (and her own, I imagine). Over the space of a critical couple of hours, with the mother of all battles raging in the victim's body, fate was settled. Either he or she expired, or the immune system suddenly got the upper hand (like an arm wrestling contest, where the loser suddenly gives in).

In which case the fever peaks, the patient stirs, opens their eyes in confusion and draws their first free breath for what seems like a month (actually less than 12 hours, usually).

Those were the days when you simply had few resources. The important thing was not to get the infections in the first place.

Well, I 'm telling you all this, not to make you feel gloomy and afraid, but to really celebrate antibiotics. They really have been one of the most, if not THE most, telling medical discovery of all time. Antibiotics have saved inestimable billions of lives.

In fact it's my firm opinion that the wonder of antibiotics is what really led us into the gullible belief that drugs were great and that there must be a chemical cure for everything. Antibiotics (and a couple of other amazing substances, like ACTH as it was prescribed then, or steroids as we prescribe them today) did seem to usher in a new era of amazing pharmaceutical cures.

Most of us are well aware that the rest of the promises of the drug industry also have not been, and will not be, fulfilled. Diseases cannot be treated as a "drug deficiency", as many doctors seem to think. It has taken decades to realize that antibiotics do not come without a price and that they will eventually fail.

The problem of this legacy today is NOT the antibiotics. It's resistance to them.

Resistance and the fact that antibiotics have made us careless; we are not nearly cautious and guarded enough of pathogens (being careful does not require being fearful, just levelheaded). Doctors and public alike have learned to be cavalier and have grown up with the attitude that antibiotics will save the day. To use antibiotics is a kind of failure; it means the important preventative basics were not being applied. Trouble is as inevitable as night follows day.

You saw the movie "Jurassic Park". You will remember Jeff Goldblum's character repeating, over and over, the warning that "Life will find a way". Life is incredibly ingenious and tough when it comes to surviving; it will get round almost any barrier, just as the dinosaurs engineered their way round an amino acid deficiency that was supposed to keep them infertile [OK, I don't normally use fictional sources—but this movie made a very important and valid scientific point].

Well—here's the thing—bacteria (and viruses and parasites, for that matter) are also life forms! They too are tough, very ingenious and swift to adapt their abilities to their needs. So in the course of time they have developed new metabolic tricks, so that antibiotics cease to work.

Man then developed newer and deadlier antibiotics. But pretty soon organisms started to adapt to those too. It's been a war of attrition. Unfortunately, Man is showing every sign of eventually losing this war. We are running out of ideas for new drugs to kill pathogens, without killing the patient.

Pathogens, it seems, will never run out of ideas to counter our efforts.

So the outcome was never in doubt. It's just that armies of irresponsible doctors have hastened the whole end by assiduously prescribing antibiotics when they are not necessary. Add to that the fact that antibiotics are used in various agricultural processes, treating livestock to enhance their growth, so the food chain is also a risk in creating antibiotic resistance.

See, the more times pathogens are exposed to toxic antibiotics, the more likely it is—just on the law of averages—that sooner or later one of them would figure out a way round the antibiotic.

As soon as a resistant strain emerges, obviously that bacterium can multiply unchallenged by therapy. Bacteria are capable of dividing every 20 minutes or so. That means in just 10 hours a single bacterium could become 268,000,000—enough to fill a bucket (at 10 hours and 20 minutes, they would divide and fill 2 buckets!) Of course this won't happen in real life, because the food supply wouldn't keep up with demand. But you get the idea? What was once just a few lucky cells, pretty soon becomes a torrent of billions, then gazillions of cells. MRSA, the hospital resistant staphylococcus, was once just such a handful of cells. Now this dreaded organism is in almost every ward in every hospital; on people's skin; in their nostrils; on their towels and clothing... just about EVERYWHERE.

That's why there is a problem.

#9 Agribusiness is to blame

It's true that doctors have abused antibiotics for decades. But the really guilty party and the truly reckless fools are those in the agribusiness (big shot farmers, livestock merchants, food manufacturers and all their hangers on).

Did you know that 70% of all antibiotic consumption goes, not to hospitals for administration to humans, but the farmers, to feed their livestock? That's according to a careful study by the Union of Concerned Scientists — and that is the main reason we're seeing the rise of pathogens that defy antibiotics.

While doctors are being urged not to use prophylactic antibiotics, even to protect human babies, farmers use them in huge quantities to protect baby calves, pigs and poultry. It's worse than criminal. It's INSANE.

It inevitably gives rise to resistant strains of bacteria, as you have learned. But these resistant, dangerous bugs don't just hang out in the farmyard! They turn up in our food supply! We swallow them!

According to Pultizer prize winning New York Times writer Nicholas Kristof , "Five out of 90 samples of retail pork in Louisiana tested positive for MRSA — an antibiotic-resistant staph infection — according to a peer-reviewed study published in Applied and Environmental Microbiology last year.

"Another recent study of retail meats in the Washington, D.C., area found MRSA in one pork sample, out of 300, according to Jianghong Meng, the University of Maryland scholar who conducted the study.

"Regardless of whether the bacteria came from the pigs or from humans who handled the meat, the results should sound an alarm bell, for MRSA already kills more than 18,000 Americans annually, more than AIDS does. A new strain called ST398 is emerging and seems to find a reservoir in modern hog farms. Research by Peter Davies of the University of Minnesota suggests that 25 percent to 39 percent of American hogs carry MRSA." Public health experts worry that pigs could pass on the infection by direct contact with their handlers, through their wastes leaking into ground water (one study has already found antibiotic-resistant bacteria entering ground water from hog farms), or through their meat, though there has been no proven case of someone getting it from eating pork.

Thorough cooking will kill the bacteria, but people often use the same knife to cut raw meat and then to chop vegetables. Or they plop a pork chop on a plate, cook it and then contaminate it by putting it back on the original plate.

Yet the central problem here isn't pigs, it's humans. Unlike Europe and even South Korea, the United States still bows to agribusiness interests by permitting the non-therapeutic use of antibiotics in animal feed. That's unconscionable.

The peer-reviewed Medical Clinics of North America ran an article last year that concluded that antibiotics in livestock feed were "a major component" in the rise in antibiotic resistance. The article said that more antibiotics were fed to animals in North Carolina alone than were administered to the nation's entire human population.

"We don't give antibiotics to healthy humans," said Robert Martin, who led a Pew Commission on industrial farming that examined antibiotic use. "So why give them to healthy animals just so we can keep them in crowded and unsanitary conditions?"

The answer is simple: greed.

Legislation to ban the non-therapeutic use of antibiotics in agriculture has always been blocked by agribusiness interests, a rich and very powerful lobby.

Louise Slaughter of New York, who is the sole microbiologist in the House of Representatives, said she planned to reintroduce the legislation this coming week. "We're losing the ability to treat humans," she said. "We have misused one of the best scientific products we've had."

That's an almost universal view in the public health world. The Infectious Diseases Society of America has declared antibiotic resistance a "public health crisis" and recounts the story of Rebecca Lohsen, a 7-year-old New Jersey girl who died from MRSA in 2006. She came down with what she thought was a sore throat, endured months in the hospital, and finally died because the microbes were too virulent for the drugs.

Again, let Nicholas Kristof speak: "This will be an important test for President Obama and his agriculture secretary, Tom Vilsack. Traditionally, the Agriculture Department has functioned mostly as a protector of agribusiness interests, but Mr. Obama and Mr. Vilsack have both said all the right things about looking after eaters as well as producers.

"So Mr. Obama and Mr. Vilsack, will you line up to curb the use of antibiotics in raising American livestock? That is evidence of an industrial farming system that is broken: for the sake of faster-growing hogs, we're empowering microbes that endanger our food supply and threaten our lives".

#10 Turning back the clock

Surgeons had a whole different attitude to infections in days past. They talked of healing by first intention and second intention. They knew how to nurse an abscess into discharging safely. These were MAJOR skills because if you got it wrong and it went to septicemia, you were likely dead.

But there were many bad problems. You wouldn't want to go back to those days. For example, cavernous sinus thrombosis. What that means is an abscess forming in the veins of the base of the brain (the cavernous sinus) and this can happen because of wounds or infected sores or spots on the head and face. Typically, the infection would travel backwards through into the skull, because there are no valves in these veins.

The cavernous sinus would sludge up and clot and the whole mass become a seething mass of infection. As a result, the brain could also become infected, a brain abscess form and death was the usual result.

That's why concerned parents of old would urge their children not to pick spots on the face and I had many a slap from my mother for trying to do so. I thought it was silly—till I went to med school years later and learned where this ancient injunction came from.

Country people didn't know much medicine but they had learned, over the centuries, that a spot around your face could kill you if it went wrong.

Teeth Infections

One of the biggest dangers of death by infection was a tooth abscess, as I wrote about in my book Virtual Medicine. At the beginning of the 20th century, the single biggest predictor of whether you are likely to die of heart disease, was teeth. You could die of a coronary, but you could die of a disastrous heart disease caused by bacteria getting loose in your blood and settling on the valves in your heart.

And of course it is not confined to the heart; bacteria that are thrown off from the teeth can travel to the brain, the kidneys and other organs.

According to one informed dentist, if we were to spread tooth infections all together on to our skin, we would have a huge infected ulcer as large as the back of our hand. Yet because this is all hidden around the roots of teeth, we ignore it and don't take the danger seriously enough.

We make light of a visit to the dentist these days, we've got used to not living with these dangers, but believe me these were very serious matters and a lot of people found themselves sick unto death quite unexpectedly, and there were many, many tragedies.

If we lose the control of microbes that antibiotics promised, we will be back in a primitive era when even the simplest health problem COULD turn out to be a fatal event.

One day, everything changed.

Along came sulphonamides. They were pretty toxic substances but the benefits far outweighed their harm.

Then penicillin arrived. It is probably the most wonderful medical breakthrough ever discovered. It has saved billions of lives. Yet penicillin remains one of the most non-toxic drugs in the entire medical armoury. It's virtually harmless (allergy is the only real problem).

Penicillin was literally a miracle. It transformed the medical landscape. For a time it looked like medical science was actually going to conquer the world.

Nobody ever considered this idea that we could go backwards; that we might lose this wonder therapy; that it could be misused and start messing up our bodies. Nobody saw that far.

Today we know that so-called "broad spectrum" antibiotics, which kill just about everything, can lead to disastrous upset of the whole bacterial colony which lives on and in our bodies. The fact that we so much depend for our health on this entire set of organisms (as described in section #2) means that antibiotics, as often as not, end up causing chronic disease; not fixing it. We call this condition dysbiosis (dys- means "bad" as in dyslexia, bad words; dysentery, bad guts; dyspepsia, bad digestion).

But of course, if you've got pneumonia, and you might die within two to three days without treatment, you are not going to care much about whether it upsets the fine balance your intestinal flora.

The real crime was the abuse of antibiotics for trivial conditions, that would self-resolve anyway. Patients became demanding and doctors became lazy and inattentive of medical basics. But there were other serious mistakes made...

One of the worst abuses was the way the STDs are treated (sexually transmitted diseases; formerly called venereal disease). It has traditionally been very difficult to treat and monitor STD cases. The shame and embarrassment mean that patients will often not re-attend for further treatment and follow up, even when strongly urged to do so, in their own interests.

Knowing this, STD clinics eventually took to trying to eradicate the infections with one-off huge doses of antibiotic.

Trouble was inevitable.

We now have antibiotic resistant gonorrhea.

Then there is resistant syphilis. This started out in the far east, with the Vietnam war. It isn't yet widespread. But it's ominous. Because if syphilis comes back as it once was, it was among the most feared diseases in civilization. Not a nice way to die. Many famous people have died of syphilis, including King Henry VIII, Schubert the composer, Lenin, Christopher Columbus and quite a few Popes by all accounts. But that's another story.

Serves them right, some people might say. That would be unkind but what about children born with this infection? It's not their fault.

Chlamydia is an organism recognized as mainly sexually transmitted and is the commonest infection in women here in the US. So it's not a time to get supercilious or puritanical. It's just the way things are.

Now in my medical school days there was a saying about syphilis. Among the many damaging effects is the fact that it attacks the main vessel from the heart and leads to deadly aneurisms. So the saying was that "The chickens of an intemperate youth come home to roost in a middle-age aorta".

Ironically, Chlamydia also attacks blood vessels, causing coronary artery inflammation and thrombosis. So we might, perhaps, modernize the saying to: The chickens of an intemperate youth come home to roost in middle-aged coronary arteries!

I'm not just being flippant. These jokey-type sayings often help memorize aspects of the data.

It was not always mistaken usage. To a certain extent, antibiotic resistance was inevitable, even given proper usage. It was just a matter of time. In fact it came very early in the 1950s. A hospital in Japan had an outbreak of Shigella, the bacterial form of dysentery. The organism was found to be multiple drug-resistant (MDR that's another term you'll hear more about) and could not be controlled by sulfonamides, chloramphenicol, tetracyclines or streptomycin.

It sent shock waves through the scientific community.

But of course it isn't just the fault of doctors. Worldwide very many antibiotics have been freely available over the counter and been taken by people who have no idea of the correct use of these powerful medicines. This is all to support sales and profits of the pharmaceutical industry and has nothing to do with medical best-practise.

Drug resistant TB is also on the rise, especially in inner cities. It's often a disease of poor people because they don't eat properly and TB is mainly a disease of malnutrition.

The overall number of tuberculosis (TB) cases in Texas has declined during the past few years, but the rate of multidrug-resistant (MDR) cases has increased, making treatment more difficult. These findings were presented at the 135th annual meeting of the American Public Health Association.

The most recent national data (2005) showed 124 of 10,662 tuberculosis cases as being MDR-TB; resistant to both the main treatment drugs. The rate is higher in immigrants.

Texas ranks second in the United States in terms of number of TB cases, after California, while New York has slipped to third, and Florida is fourth.

Even if treatment is successful it takes a LONG time. The average time to complete therapy for a drug-resistant case is a year; it doubles to 2 years for MDR-TB, while some individuals can take up to 3 years to rid themselves of the disease. Most treatment is conducted as directly observed therapy (DOT). The patient is watched, to ENSURE that he or she swallows it!

Part 2

What Can You Do To Kill Bacteria?

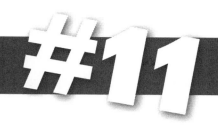

Let's start with simple remedies first. What's cheap, plentiful, non-patented and very effective for eliminating bacteria? Chlorhexidine? Dettol? Give up?

It's water. Plain water, not saline. Plain water, not antiseptic scrub even! That's according to a study published in January 2008.

Don't forget, water is very cleansing. It can dilute toxins and wash away toxins and organisms. That will help the body fight infection. Doctors, pharmacies and hospitals use saline, which is a salt solution at the same concentration as the body tissues. This is gentler. But at a pinch, water will do fine. In fact just as well and is much cheaper, of course. If it's healthy enough to drink, it's healthy enough to use on an open wound is the basic message from a recent extensive study, published in the Cochrane Database of Systematic Reviews, January 24, 2008.

The results might seem surprising: compared with hospital saline, tap water was more effective in reducing the infection rate in adults with acute wounds but not in children. To me that evens out at about the same. No real difference in other words.

There were lots of easy criticisms of the methodology used in this study. Some of the comparisons were based on a single trial. But I don't think the little details detract from the main overall finding: water works just fine. Besides, drugs get into the market place at huge profits with far less credible science than this.

Although wound care has changed significantly in the last decade, there has been limited focus on the types of solutions used for wound cleansing. Antiseptic preparations have been traditionally used, but animal models suggest that antiseptics may actually hinder healing.

Saline irrigation has been the natural alternative for doctors. But plain water is just fine for the rest of us.

No getting away from it: washing your hands is a good protection against the transmission of germs. I have already pointed out to you that it won't protect you against the pneumonic form of MRSA. But the likelihood of transmitting almost any other bacteria, including the regular MRSA, is proven to be reduced.

Heck, this was the story told over a century ago by Ignaz Semmelweiss. He pointed out that if surgeons would just wash their hands after dissecting dead bodies and BEFORE they put their fingers into the intimate parts of women in labor, that dreaded childbed fever (puerperal sepsis) was virtually eliminated.

Since this fever had almost 100% mortality, you would think doctors would rejoice in the discovery. But in fact they attacked Semmelweiss with such a fury and vengeance that the poor man eventually committed suicide. Thus passed one of my great heroes and a medical giant, brought down by ignorant pygmies.

But his message remains clear and bright. Hand washing is good; dirty hands and fingers, bad.

Antibiotic Soap?

Contrary to what you may think, antibiotic soaps are a BAD idea. They are not only not necessary, they may contribute to the development of antibiotic-resistant strains, which is definitely a bad thing.

Despite the proven health benefits of hand washing, many people don't practice this habit as often as they should — even after using the toilet. If you don't wash your hands frequently enough, you can infect yourself with these germs by touching your eyes, nose or mouth. And you can spread these germs to others by touching them or by touching surfaces that they also touch, such as doorknobs.

Infectious diseases that are commonly spread through hand-to-hand contact include the common cold, flu and several gastrointestinal disorders, such as infectious diarrhea. While most people will get over a cold, the flu can be much more serious. Some people with the flu, particularly older adults and people with chronic medical problems, can develop pneumonia. The combination of the flu and pneumonia, in fact, is the eighth-leading cause of death among Americans.

Inadequate hand hygiene also contributes to food-related illnesses, such as salmonella and E. coli infection. According to the Centers for Disease Control and Prevention (CDC), as many as 76 million Americans get a food-borne illness each year. Of these, about 5,000 die as a result of their illness. Others experience the annoying signs and symptoms of nausea, vomiting and diarrhea.

The moral is clear: wash 'em. And often. Sanitizers are merely an option. As I said, we don't need these. But if you must, the US Center For Disease Control (CDC) recommends choosing products that contain at least 60 percent alcohol.

To use an alcohol-based hand sanitizer:

- Apply about 1/2 teaspoon of the product to the palm of your hand.

- Rub your hands together, covering all surfaces of your hands, until they're dry.

If your hands are visibly dirty, however, wash with soap and water, if available, rather than a sanitizer.

When should you wash your hands?

- After using the toilet

- After changing a diaper — wash the diaper-wearer's hands, too

- After touching animals or animal waste

- Before and after preparing food, especially after handling raw meat or poultry

- Before eating

- After blowing your nose

- After coughing or sneezing into your hands

- Before and after treating wounds or cuts

- Before and after touching a sick or injured person

- After handling garbage

- Before inserting or removing contact lenses

- When using public restrooms, such as those in airports, train stations, etc.

Kids need clean hands, too

You can help your children avoid getting sick by insisting that they wash their hands properly and frequently. To get kids into the habit, teach by example. Wash your hands with your children and supervise their hand washing. Place hand-washing reminders at children's eye level, such as a chart by the bathroom sink for children to mark every time they wash their hands.

Make sure the sink is low enough for children to use, or that it has a stool underneath so that children can reach it. Tell your children to wash their hands for as long as it takes them to sing their ABCs, "Row, Row, Row Your Boat" or the "Happy Birthday" song. This works especially well with younger children, who may rush when washing their hands.

Hand washing doesn't take much time or effort, but it offers great rewards in terms of preventing illness. Adopting this simple habit can play a major role in protecting your health.

#12 Drawing Salve and Ointments

Here's another "golden oldy".

"Drawing" is a very ancient technique that needs to be kept in view. Sometimes it works instead of antibiotics; sometimes it needs to be used in conjunction.

It simply means to draw the fluid out of a swollen infected sore, boil, wound or abscess. A highly concentrated substances, such as icthammol or zinc oxide paste is smeared over the infected site and kept in contact with a bandage or poultice. It sucks out the moisture by the scientific principle of osmosis.

The dehydration effect has two benefits: bacteria don't like it, it sucks moisture from them and they die (that's the principle of using a strong sugar density in jelly, jam and conserves). But it also draws moisture from the inflammation site, which lessens the pressure and so makes it less painful.

What was red, swollen and tense tissue turns soft, crinkly and less painful. It's a sort of halfway house to lancing a boil or abscess; reducing the pressure without needing to actually make a cut.

Very often the use of a drawing salve alone will eradicate an unpleasant boil or infection resulting from a splinter or small wound. But beware: it does not remove diseases which make skin infections a hazard, such as diabetes or compromised immunity.

One of the simplest is 25% zinc oxide paste, from the regular pharmacopeia. It is readily available in small tubes or tins.

Close favorite is 20% icthammol ointment or "black drawing salve". It stinks and looks unpleasant—but it does the job. Herbs such as Calendula, Echinacea and others in a base of beeswax and Vitamin E or olive oil may be added to the icthammol salve. Cover with a bandage since it stains clothing.

Hylands Homeopathic Drawing Salve: An oldie but a goodie, Hylands (also called PRID Drawing Salve) includes components of both a drawing salve and homeopathic remedy. Eight physicians invented this salve in 1903. PRID contains the homeopathic ingredient acidum carbolicum along with herbs such as calendula and Echinacea. Other ingredients include ichthammol, sulphur and silicea.

At a pinch you can make your own drawing salve, using the strongest solution you can make of table salt or Epsom salts in hot water. Soak a bandage or compress in the mixture and then apply. Unfortunately, this remedy needs frequent repeat applications over many hours.

You could also try a lavender and tea tree oil compress: Both lavender and tea tree oil contain antibacterial agents particularly useful against boils (see section #39).

Drop tea tree oil directly onto the boil for one to two days during the first phases to bring it quickly to a head. Lavender, however, is too irritating for direct application.

Margosa or Neem is a very effective natural antibiotic. You can make an ointment for boils by boiling some neem seeds in water till they are soft. Then take some neem leaves and smash them to make a pulp. Mix these boiled neem seeds and neem leaves and you get a natural ointment for boils which can be directly applied to the area. Moreover this poultice even prevents the infection from spreading as well.

You can even use castor ointment for boils. All you need to do is to make a powder out of the castor bark and add some water to turn it into a paste. You can even add grind the root of the herb biskhapra for additional effect.

Another effective ointment for boils can be made by grinding onion and garlic paste. This can aid in healing the boil quickly.

Always wash your hands thoroughly after treating boils. The bacteria spread easily from person to person, and can spread from one area of the body to another.

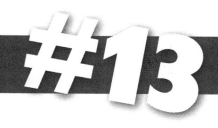

#13 Blue light

Next comes a pretty simple method of sterilization from the world of physics. Light.

One of the miracles of the amazing electromagnetic spectrum, which I explain to people is the fact that although most of the electromagnetic spectrum is very hostile to life (such as microwaves, ultraviolet light, and gamma rays), the fact is that a very narrow band of the electromagnetic spectrum, that we call "light" is not only friendly, but is actually essential to life.

However, here is a useful reminder that even light is part of that dangerous spectrum, and can have destructive effects on living organisms, blue light especially (red light, which spills over into the infrared range is warmth, and therefore also somewhat supportive of life).

Blue light, being close to the ultraviolet range, can itself be quite harmful, and we can cash in on this property and make it useful. We find the bluelight is great for killing resistant bacteria, as a study published in Photomedicine and Laser Surgery, April 2009, shows.

Specifically, blue light NOT including dangerous UV frequencies, kills MRSA (see section 45 for news about the safe use of UV light as an antibiotic).

The finding comes from Chukuka S. Enwemeka, PhD, and colleagues at New York Institute of Technology. Their study was funded by Dynatronics Corp., which makes the blue-light device used in the study.

In earlier studies, Enwemeka's team found that MRSA died when exposed to blue light that included part of the ultraviolet (UV) spectrum. Even though the total UV dose was less than that of a few minutes of sunlight, it would be safer not to expose humans to any more UV light than necessary.

So the researchers used a LED device that emits only blue light, not UV, and found it worked nearly as well!

"Irradiation with [blue] light energy may be a practical, inexpensive alternative to treatment with pharmacologic agents, particularly in cases involving cutaneous and subcutaneous MRSA infections," Enwemeka and colleagues conclude. The researchers tested two MRSA strains: one typical of the strains that bedevil hospitals, and one typical of the strains found in the community. Both strains were susceptible to the blue light.

Relatively low doses of blue light, less than 2 minutes, killed off about 30% of MRSA in laboratory cultures. Obviously, longer exposure was better, but 100% death of organisms did not come about, even through very long exposures.

Exactly how blue light kills MRSA, or whether the bacteria can become blue-light resistant, isn't known.

Tell your doctor about this study if you get any resistant surface infection. But remember also, light penetrates well below the skin layer (shine a torch through your hand on a dark night and you will see what I mean).

See just how valuable light is by viewing this YouTube video by Dr. John Ott, one of the pioneers in light and health (I featured his work in Virtual Medicine, first published 1999).

http://www.youtube.com/watch?v=bw6hcTGND3c

And let me close by commenting that fresh air and sunlight have traditionally been recognized for their healing powers. Moms always knew it! To expose an infected wound to bright sunlight would do far more good than covering it with bandages, most especially if the organism is one of these resistant toughies anyway.

I always do away with the band aid at the earliest available moment, for this reason.

Get a UV Light Nano To Protect Yourself Against Dangerous Bacteria

Note: You can always get a Nano UV germ zapper. It's a handy electronic gardget that looks like a cell phone and is about the same size. But it delivers a powerful light punch; a mixture of UV-A, UV-B and UV-C.

Read more in section #47.

Soon, we are going to do some nutrition stuff. But this next few are different. It's from the larder but not quite nutrition!

Let's start with a surprising contender: HONEY! What's surprising is not that it works as an antibtioic but that conventional doctors and hospitals openly admit its efficacy!

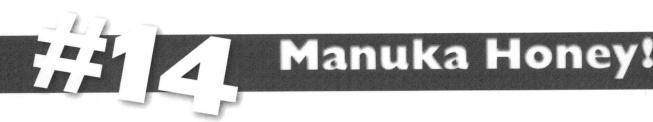

Honey has been known for its healing properties for thousands of years - the Ancient Greeks used it, and so have many other peoples through the ages. Even up to the Second World War, honey was being used for its antibacterial properties in treating wounds. Then along came antibiotics, as I explained, and it was promptly forgotten.

But in recent times there has been a renaissance of the use of honey in the medical profession: an editorial in the Journal of the Royal Society of Medicine (Zumla and Lulat 1989) discussing this expressed the opinion "The therapeutic potential of uncontaminated, pure honey is grossly underutilized".

I know for example that bandages soaked in manuka honey were given to patients at the Christie Cancer Hospital in Manchester to reduce their chances of contracting the MRSA superbug and to lessen wound inflammation following surgery.

Honey is used routinely at the Manchester Royal Infirmary for dressing wounds, and other research has found it can fight gum disease, ease digestive problems and soothe sore throats (I got my bachelor of medicine and bachelor of surgery at Manchester University and so I know the Christie and the Royal Infirmary very well).

The way honey works is that it is very rich, it is like jam or preserves you know; adding the sugar to the fruit is what makes it impossible for the bacteria to grow, it just sucks the water out of them so they can't grow and honey does the same thing. So remember diluted honey does not work and will cause bacteria to flourish!

A British team from the famous University of Oxford and the Radcliffe Hospital in Woodstock Road, Oxford (I added that for you Morse fans out there), have done a systematic review of the use of honey as a wound dressing, compared to other dressings and treatments *[BMC Complement Altern Med. 2001; 1: 2. Published online 2001 June 4. doi: 10.1186/1472-68821-2]*.

Time for healing was significantly shorter for honey than all other treatments but, the researchers complained, the quality of studies was low. However the results were pretty clear, taken over the number of studies. Honey won every time.

There was one study in which the healing of infected postoperative wounds compared honey with antiseptics in addition to systemic antibiotics after culture and sensitivity. For all outcomes honey was significantly better, with much shorter times for healing, eradication of infection, use of antibiotics and hospital stay.

[Al-Waili NS, Saloom KY. Effects of topical honey on post-operative wound infections due to Gram positive and Gram negative bacteria following Caesarean sections and hysterectomies. Eur J Med Res. 1999;4:126–30]

Another study I found in the British Journal Of Surgery (which was not included in the Oxford group review) showed dramatic benefits from honey in treating infected wounds and ulcers.

Fifty-nine patients with wounds and ulcers most of which (80 per cent) had failed to heal with conventional treatment were treated with unprocessed honey. Fifty-eight cases showed remarkable improvement following topical application of honey. Only one case, later diagnosed as Buruli ulcer, failed to respond (Buruli ulcer is caused by Mycobacterium ulcerans, a relative of TB). *[Br J Surg. 1988 Jul;75(7):679-81].*

What's especially interesting is that honey allows wound healing with little or no scarring. It seems that honey is able to restrain the excessive growth of collagen which takes place during wound healing. The less collagen, the less scarring.

[Topham J. Why do some cavity wounds treated with honey or sugar paste heal without scarring? J Wound Care. 2002 Feb;11(2):53-5].

Propolis

Propolis is the resinous substance collected by bees from the leaf buds and bark of trees, especially poplar and conifer trees. Bees use the propolis along with beeswax to construct their hives. Because of antimicrobial properties of propolis, it helps keep hives free of germs.

The great violin makers Stradivarius and Guaneri used unique blends of oils, resins, beeswax, and propolis, to varnish their instruments and no doubt protect them against mold and microorganisms.

Propolis has a long history of use in folk medicine and was even used as a conventional doctor's drug in London in the 1600s. It appears to have antimicrobial and anti-inflammatory activities. In the past, propolis has been taken by mouth to fight bacterial infection including tuberculosis, fungal infection such as Candidiasis, parasitic infections such as malaria, and viral infections such as colds.

A study published in the November 2001 of the journal Mycoses investigated the effect of propolis on 80 strains of Candida yeasts, including:

- 20 strains of Candida albicans

- 20 strains of Candida tropicalis

- 20 strains of Candida krusei and

- 15 strains of Candida guilliermondii

The yeasts showed propolis had a clear antifungal activity and was especially useful against Candida albicans.

While not conclusive evidence has yet been produced, propolis may offer a number of other health/medicinal benefits including the following:

Popolis contains a special compound which may interfere with inflammatory messengers in the body. This potential effect may help to relieve inflammatory conditions such as arthritis.

Propolis may enhance the function of the immune system.

A few studies have shown some activity against cancer cells.

Several other laboratory studies found that propolis may protect the liver from damage by alcohol or environmental toxins.

A recent study of individuals with second-degree burns, compared propolis cream and a prescription burn cream and showed the two were about comparable in preventing infection. But propolis cream promoted earlier healing and seemed to decrease inflammation more than the prescription cream. (I would use homeopathic calendula cream, for burns).

Other studies have also shown that an alcohol-based mouth rinse of propolis may help eliminate oral bacteria: those that can cause dental cavities, gingivitis, and periodontal disease.

For instance, a 1996 study tested the antibacterial properties of propolis and honey against oral bacteria. The antibacterial effects of propolis and honey on oral streptococci were determined using bacterial culture plates. The researchers also clinically checked the short-term antibacterial effect of propolis solution and honey on salivary total bacteria and Streptococcus mutans was tested in 10 volunteers.

Propolis demonstrated an antibacterial effect both in vitro on isolated oral streptococci and in the clinical study on salivary bacterial counts. Honey induced bacteria growth at low concentrations, while at high concentrations honey had an inhibitory effect on bacterial growth in vitro.

Salivary counts of total bacteria and Streptococcus mutans were lower for 1 hour after application of honey.

[Steinberg D; Kaine G; Gedalia I, Antibacterial effect of propolis and honey on oral bacteria. American Journal Of Dentistry 1996;9(6):236-9].

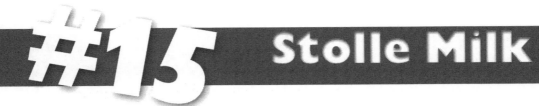

This is something that's really useful to know, when antibiotics have run out. Talking about cheap!

Suppose there existed a cheap, safe, widely available effective oral "vaccine" that was:

- 100% safe for all who use it;

- can be taken orally and tastes good;

- can be manufactured in virtually every country in the world, with the humble technology available to many third-world nations;

- so cheap that virtually everyone in the world can afford it;

- able to protect against a wide variety of organisms, including viruses, rickettsia, parasites, protozoan, bacteria, mycoplasm, yeast/fungus, amoeba;

- capable of reducing or eliminating allergic reactions to vast numbers of exogenous and endogenous substances;

- boosts the immune system, accelerates healing of injuries, helps repair nervous system damage, burns fat and builds lean muscle, increases vitality and stamina, and elevates mood;

- and might – just might – deal a deadly blow against a number of cancers?

Suppose, moreover, there were over 4,000 clinical studies worldwide which describe the efficacy of this oral vaccine in the treatment of hundreds of different infectious diseases.

Would you be interested to know what it was?

I'll bet you would.

It's milk protein concentrate. Why do I call it an oral vaccine? Well, that's the really interesting part. Let Anthony di Fabio take up the story:

"Bessie, our former pet milk cow, lived in a small pasture of not more than three acres. She munched on uncooked grasses during the summer and uncooked dry hay during the winter, licked mineral block, and drank from a rain-filled, surface-drained pond whose waters were loaded with a wide variety of microorganisms. The pond also held frogs, snakes, bugs, worms, snails, and so on. She often drank and urinated at the same time, recycling fluids from the pond even as she drank.

When she was ready to drop her calf, we led her to an old barn that had held forty head of cattle. One's nose almost stifled from sediments of dust, mold, fungi, and dried manure layered fifty years deep. When Bessie's calf, Nina (pronounced "Neenya"), was born, she lacked effective defensive mechanisms against the blizzard of microorganisms that assailed her in every cubic inch of the air she breathed, the ground she stood on, or on the inexperienced tongue she extended to various surfaces. Almost by magic, thousands of potentially deadly microorganisms invaded her immature body.

Nina, as with all calves, was also born with a leaky gut! Now pay attention here, because I know that many readers have a leaky gut, a condition where the stomach lining is so thin that whole, undigested protein molecules pass directly from the stomach into the blood stream. Once inside the bloodstream these protein molecules are identified as foreign invaders, and we create antibodies to counteract them. This situation brings about food allergies.

Patients and their doctors both work very, very hard to get rid of the patient's leaky gut. Their leaky gut is considered the source of many degenerative diseases – or at least a major component of them. But Bessie and Nina had found a way to make the leaky gut a beneficial survival mechanism! When Nina wobbled to her feet and gently nudged at Bessie's milk sac, the very first milk to come was colostrum. As Nina prodded the milk sac with her nose and sucked as saliva dripped, she also injected her blizzard of rapidly multiplying microorganisms into Bessie's teat, and up into Bessie's milk sac into a portion called the "'cistern."

Inside Bessie's cistern specialized cells that had been lying dormant came alive, and they started manufacturing – guess what? – "disease-specific antibodies," and immune-boosting "complement," and also flooding her cistern with "immunoglobulins" and "growth factors"!

Very shortly after Nina introduced her stream of potentially dangerous microorganisms into Bessie's teat – then into Bessie's cistern – her mammary biochemical factory stimulated specialized cells that became active and began to create disease-specific antibodies and activated complement that mingled with Nina's first fluids, the colostrum, which Nina sucked back into her leaky gut from Bessie's teats. Bessie was generating vaccines for her calf!

The immunoglobulins, growth factors and these disease-specific antibodies and their helpers, the complement, passed directly into Nina's stomach, and there they attached themselves to whatever corresponding organisms were present inside the gut, killing many. Because of Bessie's leaky gut many of these specially prepared biological agents also passed directly into Nina's bloodstream, and within her blood plasma they attached themselves to whatever microorganisms they'd been designed to destroy and killed them. Never once was Nina placed in danger from the surrounding hostile environment whose every biological niche was filled with a wide variety of deadly microorganisms.

Milk is thus the ideal vaccine! At least dedicated and immune-competent milk is.

According to Herbert Struss, PhD, former Senior Chemist, Food Chemistry Laboratory, Minnesota Department of Agriculture Laboratory Services Division – and also a scientist who was involved in much of the early clinical work testing this wondrously universal vaccine – those interested in "immune milk" (as it is called) during the '60s, made their astounding oral vaccine discoveries when they were trying to answer the question: "What's the survival advantage to being a mammal?"

All animals evolve traits that persist because they have a survival advantage. So what is the advantage to being a mammal? (a mammal, remember, defines a creature with teats or "mammary glands", hence the name) Clearly, Nina's suckling at Bessie's teat, drawing a blood-like liquid called "colostrum" from Bessie's cistern was a possible answer to their question. The survival advantage was simply that an "acquired" or "adaptive" immunity could be transferred from mother to offspring and that this adaptive immunity would extend for some period of time, thus providing the offspring with a distinct survival advantage.

Human milk may not have quite the same importance for survival, as it is with multilayered placentas such as horse, goats, and cattle. But some immunity does pass from the mother to the human child. It is obvious that a breast-fed human baby usually has an advantage over bottle fed. Breast-fed infants have a far lower incidence of early disease and also allergies.

They have been vaccinated by Nature, through nurture. Colostrum is a very special form of milk immune concentrate. See the next section.

But we will continue with our discussion of milk protein concentrate or "hyper-immune milk", as it is known. Thousands of good scientific papers have been published on its power immune properties. We can start the story with Drs. Wlliam "Pete" Peterson, Barry Campbell, and other colleagues working at the University of Minnesota from 1950 to 1958. They used killed bacterial antigens injected into the teat of a cow (ouch!!) and collected the first ten days' colostrum. Peterson's interest was in treating rheumatoid arthritis and allergies, which he did successfully.

In the late 1950s a wealthy businessman called Ralph Stolle, owner-operator of the San-MarGale Farm in Lebanon (Ohio), stepped into the picture. Stolle took an interest in hyper-immune milk, simply as a hobby. He developed a better way of using the cow to provoke a beneficial antigen response, by injecting pathogens into the cow's bloodstream and then harvesting the milk. Using his personal fortune he gave out thousands of portions of hyper-immune milk and asked the users to report back its benefits. Over a total of some 35 years a total of 8000 people reported a variety of benefits, from joint pain relief (85%) to improvement in fatigue (74%) and lowering cholesterol (71%). This series probably constitutes one of the largest open clinical trials ever carried out.

Stolle went into partnership with the New Zealand Dairy Board to make very pure hyperimmune milk concentrate or "Stolle milk" as it was known. In 1988 it went on sale in Asia for the first time. It is freeze dried and shipped to third world countries, where it is a very valuable vaccination and therapy resource. It can also be rendered homeopathically, so that the cost is even less. In 1999 Spencer Trask purchased Stolle Milk Biologics Inc (SMBI).

It seems to me there is an important dimension that has been missed for decades. The family cow was the manufacturer of home-grown vaccines for humans. Folks lived mainly in a rural environment and milked their own beasts. Not just landowners; even farm workers had access to a Bessie-type vaccine factory. The cow would be infected with all present human pathogens, make antibodies and give these back in the milk.

That's why most of those country folks were so darned healthy, I believe. They had a constant supply of free and effective personalized vaccines down on the farm. Far better than modern vaccine attempts manufactured in a test tube and under the pretense that everyone is in the same circumstance and health status.

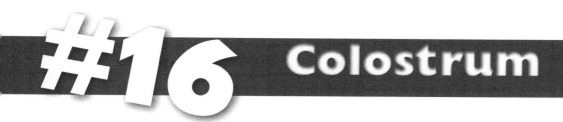

Milk brings me to colostrum, the thin yellowish fluid secreted by the mammary glands at the time of parturition that is rich in antibodies and minerals, and precedes the production of true milk. It is also called foremilk.

Mother's colostrum, incidentally, is vitally important to human babies. It transfers mother's immunity to infection to the child and protects it for the first few weeks of life. There are no antibodies, of course, in milk formulas.

Commercial colostrum is produced by cows that were previously vaccinated with certain kind of pathogens. These cows will then produce antibodies in their blood and then transferred them to milk they produced, just like hyperimmune milk. But the highest concentration of antibodies is transferred in Colostrum, the first drops expressed from the teat.

According to research data, there are around 90 known immunologically-active substances in colostrum, including growth factors, lipids, lactoferrin (iron-binding protein with antimicrobial qualities), cytokines [released from T cells, they inhibit replication of viruses and chemicals (cytotoxins) that kill the infected cell], etc.

Immune Factors in colostrum have been shown to help the body fight off harmful invaders such as viruses, bacteria, yeast and fungus. Each factor plays a specific role in our body's defense against these attackers. In addition, colostrum contains over 20 antibodies to specific pathogens including E coli, salmonella, rotavirus, candida, streptococcus, staphylococcus, H pylori, and cryptosporidia.

In addition to immunoglobulins, medical studies show that PRP in colostrum also supports an under active immune system. Some workers say it has great benefit in treating cancer immunologically. PRP also helps balance an overactive immune system present in autoimmune diseases.

A 2003 study by the Health Sciences Department of the University of South Australia suggests that taking concentrated bovine colostrum supplements could reduce the incidence of respiratory tract infections. The study involved subjects being randomly allocated to consume 60g/day of Colostrum for eight weeks, then examining their occurrence of symptoms. Results from the first week were kept separate from those from the last seven weeks.

The results showed that during the first week of supplementation, there was no measurable difference in symptoms in the proportion of subjects taking the supplement as opposed to those who didn't. During the subsequent seven weeks, however, a much lower percentage of the subjects taking Colostrum reported upper respiratory infection related symptoms.

Symptom duration, however, did not differ. This suggests that the immune benefits achieved by Colostrum can be very good in terms of being a preventative, but that it does not have any measurable effect on an infection once it has already taken hold. That is why it is important to use Colostrum properly, as a preventative, and not depend on it to cure illness.

Another study by Susanna Rokka of MTT Agrifood Research Finland, showed the same thing, testing the ability of Bovine Colostrum to help fight Helicobacter Pylori infections. Helicobacter is a kind of bacteria that is often responsible for Gastritis, Gastric ulcer, and Stomach Cancer.

The research also showed that immune milk combined with lactobacilli that's extracted from fermented cabbage can effectively help in preventing Streptococcus and Helicobacter Pylori. Streptococcus is the most responsible bacteria in causing dental caries from adhering to tooth surface.

So, logically, it makes sense to take colostrum (60 gr daily) alongside whatever alternative antibiotic treatment you are engaged in. What we English call "belt and braces" (I suppose for Americans it would be belt and suspenders).

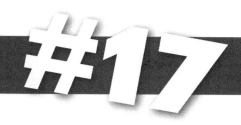

Shockingly, I only got to know of Quinton recently, while staying at Dr. Garry Gordon's home. He'd only just found it too. My ignorance was despite years of practice in Europe, where Quinton has been big business in the healing arts for over a century. A well kept secret, you might say.

What is Quinton? Sea water!

Well, not just any old sea water. It's special vortex water from certain blooms in the oceans, that are very rich in nutrients. It seems to have energetic properties too, above and beyond the mere presence of rare minerals etc.

Let me back up a tad, before we come to the product. The floor of our oceans is indescribably rich in minerals. Think about this: EVERYTHING that ever lived and died goes into the water system, down the rivers and ultimately finds its way to the ocean. Added to that is all the ocean life which lives, dies and is recycled, all the plankton, corals, fish, feces, EVERYTHING, which falls to the ocean floor as organic debris.

There is thick mud at the bottom of the ocean that contains dense nutrients and some minerals that are otherwise incredibly rare, like iridium, osmium, yttrium and so on.

But it doesn't just stay on the ocean bed, lost to the biosystem. Quite the contrary. This nourishing mud is carried around the ocean floor by submarine currents which have only recently begun to be understood. There are certain places where this nutrient deposit wells up to the surface. Giant surges of ocean currents that we call convergences stir up the seas and bring the nutrients back to the bio system.

The polar oceans are classic sites for this. The huge bloom of algae that takes place in the Arctic and Antarctic every year yields a staggering abundance of life where the ocean, literally, changes color due to the density of life it carries. Waters turn red with krill and other plankton.

This bloom is so rich it feeds the greatest animals of all: the whales. So much nutrition is absorbed into the biosystem at these sites in the summer time that whales can double their weight and deposit enough fat or blubber to live on it through the winter months.

But there are the birds, fishes and other animals too, so that the polar oceans literally burst with life every spring when the returning sun ignites the nutrition chain. Given the right wind and currents, then these blooms can be carried far and wide. Scientists report this year there has been a huge upsurge in nutrients and an explosion of sea life off Monterrey, California, from currents brought all the way down from the Arctic.

The polar regions are not the only upsurges, however. In fact they can take place anywhere, if the wind blows the water out to sea; then underwater currents draw up deeper water to fill the gap.

That's what I mean by ocean nutrients, OK?

Enter Messieur Rene Quinton...

Rene Quinton (pronounced cahn-ton) was a Frenchman, a doctor, biologist, biochemist and physiologist. He discovered the healing merits of marine plankton plasma, drawn from deep ocean water upsurges, right at the end of the nineteenth century. It is a little known fact that by 1907 Quinton had established 69 Marine Dispensaries and the product was already saving countless lives throughout the deadly pandemics of the early 20th century (tuberculosis, typhoid, cholera, syphilis, influenza).

When Quinton was finally buried in 1925, his fame had reached such proportions that tens of thousands of men, women and children, not to mention generals, dignitaries and statesmen, attended the funeral. Yet we have never heard of him. How can that be?

Think "Pharma" and think "eliminating the competition", no matter how good the product. The stark truth is I never heard of this cure, all through my medical training. No libraries have editions of his work; no pharmacy has heard of it; no learning institutions teach it. He's been deleted! Especially in his native France.

Quinton's marine plasma (or QMP) was considered so effective for a wide range of common afflictions that is was reimbursed under two French laws, including Social Security. It was, of course, absurdly cheap. But that didn't suit the drug barons, who wanted to peddle their costly and dangerous garbage for huge profits. Through their bribes and malign abuse they got a law passed, requiring QMP to be heat treated. That would effectively ruin its properties and so put Quinton out of business.

However, Quinton manufacture did not fold up. The operation was moved to Spain instead.

Thanks to the more liberal scientific climate in Spain it has survived until today.

Now QMP has arrived in the US and is being sold by Original Quinton of Buena Park, CA.

Properties of QMP

As I write this I have in front of me a translation of the entry for Quinton Marine Plasma in the French Medical Dictionary of 1975 (a kind of PDR). It describes the product as a sterile apyrogenic solution (pH 7.2) of seawater, prepared under aseptic conditions by special processes without rise in temperature or exposure to electric potential or field, in order to preserve its molecular balance and its character as an "alive medium".

The seawater is extracted from a 30-metre depth (zone of solar penetration) under special conditions and from special locations.

It contains 92 elements of the periodic table (all primary and trace minerals).

The entry goes on to add "Rene Quinton showed, in 1904, that QUINTON MARINE PLASMA is identical physically, chemically, and physiologically, to our interior milieu (extracellular fluid) and provides optimum conditions for red blood corpuscles and leucocytes and other blood fractions. It is possible to replace the entire blood volume of an animal with QUINTON MARINE PLASMA without any disorders for the organism." Sacrebleu! Shades of Ringer's solution!

Without any intellectual prowess, one can therefore deduce that QMP is very safe, helps stabilize the internal milieu, provides every conceivable nutrient mineral and provides low concentration homeopathic-type mechanisms for healing. It's a miracle!

Well, it isn't really. It's just Nature at her best. But you can see why Rene Quinton was adored by millions and hated by Big Pharma. Here is a substance that's cheap to manufacture, no patents, is readily available and works wonders as a natural "antibiotic".

The "indications" (reasons to use it) are manifold and include: childhood gastroenteritis, poisoning, malnutrition and eczema; anemia, asthma, exhaustion, anti-aging, dysentery, tuberculosis and atherosclerosis; uterine and vaginal infections; rhinitis, sinusitis, respiratory allergies; skin allergies, dermal infections, histaminic reactions and psoriasis; energy restoration; bioterrain restoration and burns.

The official French pharmacopeia (1975) even lists it as an "antibiotic solvent and carrier".

I have even found that dentists can use it to save teeth, by injecting this healing balm into the surrounding gums. The abcesses and periodontal disease simply disappear.

There are DOZENS more uses.

How To Take It

QMP is taken by injections or orally. When injected, there is an isotonic form, which does not sting. Orally, the full-strength version is fine.

Sprays work well for skin conditions.

It can even be taken by nebulizer, just breathed in. Or I find it very soothing for tired eyes.

Just the whiff of "sea air" is very restorative to me!

It's so safe there are no real limits on the number of ampoules. It's only body fluid, after all!

You can't OD on it like water (too much water will kill you).

QMP comes in 10 ml ampoules. 2, 3, 5, 10 ampoules are fine, depending on the seriousness of the complaint. It's so cheap, cost is not an issue (around $3 an ampoule) Note that Quinton is not FDA approved for injection in the USA.

Next we come to a modern surprise. The story of how it was discovered is interesting. One of those serendipity things!

The idea of using chlorine dioxide was developed by Jim Humble, a gold miner and metallurgist, on an expedition into the jungles of Central America, looking for gold. It was a response to a need to help a member of his expedition who came down with malaria, more than two days away, through heavy jungle, from the next mine.

After many years of experience, Humble always carried "stabilized oxygen" (sodium chlorite) with him on such expeditions, to make local water safe to drink. Facing the possibility of a quick loss of life, he gave it to the stricken man. To everyone's amazement, the patient was well within a few hours. That seemed like a miracle, but Humble wanted to better understand what had just happened.

Over the course of several years, Jim Humble figured out that what made stabilized oxygen so effective in some malaria cases, was not the oxygen at all, but the trace amounts of chlorine dioxide it contained. Further research led him to come up with a way to produce hundreds, if not thousands more units of chlorine dioxide than what is found in stabilized oxygen. This is done by using a higher concentration of sodium chlorite (28% vs. 3% for stabilized oxygen), in conjunction with an activator.

Humble went on the have great success using his new formula which, unscientifically, has been named "Magic Minerals Solution" (there are no minerals in it). But MMS (for short) does seem to work, though I doubt some of the claims. It is said to been successful in helping over 75,000 people in several African nations – including Uganda and Malawi – rid themselves, primarily of malaria, but also hepatitis, cancer, and AIDS.

Anyone can be overloaded with toxins. Most people probably are but won't admit it or, more likely, don't know it. Others would prefer to think they're not. If your health is not perfect, you're habitually low on energy, have trouble keeping your weight down or your blood pressure in the normal range, or constantly dealing with inflammation or pain, or indeed have any medical condition that is adversely affecting your health, then there's likely to be a toxin, heavy metal, virus, bacteria, fungus, or parasite playing a part. Mainstream medicine will typically respond by loading you up with additional pollutants, many of which indiscriminately kill healthy tissue while going after "the bad guys" to deal with the symptoms. Not so with chlorine dioxide. It only acts on anything harmful. Miracle or not, the effects can be amazing!

Over the next few pages, the MMS protocol will be described. When followed, it will produce and distribute chlorine dioxide to your red blood cells, which are the most effective and intelligent pathogen killers known to Nature, although your white blood cells are assumed to do all the work.

But first, a little background on the chemistry. Chlorine dioxide and chlorine are not the same. Chlorine is a chemical element. In ionic form, chlorine is part of common salt and other compounds, and is necessary to most forms of life, including human. A powerful oxidizing agent, it is the most abundant dissolved ion in ocean water, and readily combines with nearly every other element, including sodium to form salt crystals, and magnesium, as magnesium chloride. Chlorine dioxide is a chemical compound that consists of one chlorine ion bound to two ions of oxygen. Oxidizing agents are chemical compounds that readily accept electrons from "electron donors." They gain electrons via chemical reaction. This is important because relative to chlorine dioxide, all pathogens are electron donors.

Chlorine dioxide is extremely volatile. You might call it "hot tempered," but in a very beneficial way. This volatility is a key factor in chlorine dioxide's effectiveness as a pathogen destroyer. The compound is literally explosive, so explosive, it's not safe to transport in any quantity. Therefore, it is common practice to generate chlorine dioxide "on site" at the point of use. Most chlorine dioxide production is done on a scale that would prove deadly for individuals, for example, in municipal water treatment systems, where it is beginning to replace chlorine because it produces no carcinogenic by-products.

Chlorine dioxide is approved by the Environmental Protection Agency in safely removing pathogens and contaminates like anthrax. So you know it must be effective. However, the concentrations used in such applications can vary from 500 to over 6,000 parts per million (ppm), which would clearly be deadly to an individual. Using the MMS protocol you will produce chlorine dioxide around 1 ppm. You will use the MMS solution, which is safe to transport, to make nature's harmless pathogen destroyer.

The MMS solution is 25% sodium chlorite in distilled water. You can produce chlorine dioxide with a single drop, when an "activator" of vinegar, lemon juice, or a 10% solution of citric acid is added. Citric acid is recommended because of its simplicity. The natural pH of sodium chlorite is 13. Adding vinegar, lemon juice, or citric acid creates about 3 mg of unstable but still harmless chlorine dioxide.

The Process

Let's talk a bit more about how and why chlorine dioxide works by giving the immune system a new lease of life. Volatility is what makes chlorine dioxide so effective when it contacts pathogens. As we've already mentioned, chlorine dioxide is a safe and effective disinfectant in many municipal water delivery systems, hospitals, and even in bio-terrorism response. It stands to reason that chlorine dioxide would be just as effective working in the waters of the human body at the appropriate dose.

Chlorine dioxide's extreme volatility prevents pathogens from developing a resistance, mainly because when they "clash," the pathogens no longer exist. Yet, healthy cells and beneficial bacteria remain unaffected. While normal levels of oxygen in the blood cannot destroy all of the pathogens present under disease conditions, delivery of chlorine dioxide changes everything. "Halt! Surrender Your Electrons, Now!" When a chlorine dioxide ion contacts a harmful pathogen, it instantly rips up to five electrons from the pathogen, in what can be likened to a microscopic explosion... harmless to us, but terminal for pathogens. The pathogen – an electron donor – is rendered harmless due to the involuntary surrendering of its electrons to the chlorine dioxide – an electron acceptor – and the resulting release of energy. Oxidized by the chlorine ion, the former pathogen becomes a harmless salt.

This process benefits a body that has become toxic. Throughout the body, anywhere chlorine dioxide ions – transported via red blood cells – come into contact with pathogens, the pathogens give up their electrons and cease to exist.

The chlorine dioxide-armed cells only "detonate" on contact with pathogens, which include harmful bacteria, viruses, funguses, toxins, heavy metals, and parasites. All of these will have pH values that are out of the body's range of good health. They will also have a positive ionic charge. The chlorine dioxide equipped cells do not oxidize beneficial bacteria, or healthy cells, as their pH levels are 7 or above, and hold a negative ionic charge. Chlorine dioxide ions will oxidize – meaning vaporize – diseased cells... anything that is acidic, with a positive ionic charge. If the chlorine dioxide ions encounter no pathogens or other poisons, they deteriorate into table salt and in some instances, hypochlorous acid, which the body can also use.

A Pathogen Terminator

Research has proven chlorine dioxide to be much safer than chlorine, as it is selective for pathogens when used in water. Furthermore, it does not create harmful compounds from other constituents in the water as chlorine does. Numerous scientific studies have demonstrated that chlorine – part of the halogen family of elements – creates as least three carcinogenic compounds when it enters the body, principally Trihalomethanes (THMs). There has been no such evidence of harmful compounds being produced from chlorine dioxide. This is why, in 1999, the American Society of Analytical Chemists proclaimed chlorine dioxide to be the most powerful pathogen killer known to man. It has even been used to clean up after anthrax attacks.

A Journey into Chemical Alchemy

Once it is introduced into the bloodstream, chlorine dioxide performs a highly energetic acceptance of up to five electrons when it comes across any cell that is below a pH value of 7.

This means that diseased cells are essentially vaporized (i.e., "oxidized") while healthy cells are unaffected.

This is how it happens. Red blood cells that are normal carriers of oxygen throughout the body do not differentiate between chlorine dioxide and oxygen. Therefore, after you have swallowed the MMS/chlorine dioxide-rich solution, red blood cells pick up chlorine dioxide ions as they pass through the stomach wall. When the red blood cells, armed with chlorine dioxide, encounter parasites, fungi, diseased cells or anything that has a pH below 7 and a positive ionic charge, the "aliens" are destroyed along with the chlorine dioxide ion.

If the chlorine dioxide doesn't hit anything that can set it off, it will eventually deteriorate, by losing an electron or two. This will allow it to be converted into hypochlorous acid. This compound kills pathogens and even cancerous cells. Hypochlorous acid is so important that its diminished presence in the body is described medically by the term 'myeloperoxidase deficiency'. Many people are afflicted by this condition. The immune system needs a great deal more hypochlorous acid when disease is present. Facilitated by the MMS solution, chlorine dioxide delivers it in quantity.

The most salient point to know is that chlorine dioxide has 100 times more energy to do what oxygen normally does, and yet, will not harm healthy cells. By the way, if you are totally healthy and have nothing in your body that is at an acidic level below 7, there are no ill effects from taking chlorine dioxide at the appropriate dose. However, your stores of hypochlorous acid will be increased.

MMS works best to destroy pathogens that may be present in the body, when 2 or 3 mg of free chlorine dioxide are in the solution at the time it is swallowed. However, the body is supplied with chlorine dioxide in a "timed release" manner lasting about 12 hours. Be aware, that before you feel better, it is likely you will feel ill in one way or another.

Nausea

The nauseating feeling that you may possibly experience, especially if you take too big a dose, is the result of chlorine dioxide encountering and destroying a large number of pathogens. We are generally oblivious to the pathogens that are present in our bodies, but there is an increasing awareness in the medical and scientific literature of their importance to our health, or more to the point our ill health. Since they build up over time in various organs of the body, they generally affect our health slowly and cumulatively. If chlorine dioxide takes them out too suddenly, the result will be a dramatic reaction. However, the time it takes to clear the pathogens and toxins is much less than it took for them to accumulate. It has probably taken many years, possibly almost a lifetime, for some of them to accumulate.

As a person always feels unwell when they contract a case of, say, acute hepatitis, dengue fever or Lyme disease, they may continue to feel unwell for a while, in which case it will be difficult to tell whether it is the condition or the chlorine dioxide that is causing the unwell feeling. However, if the condition is treated with chlorine dioxide in its early stages, the pathogens will be killed off quickly as they are still in the blood stream and therefore available to be attacked easily by the circulating chlorine dioxide-rich red blood cells. Under these circumstances, the symptoms should be over very quickly.

In chronic conditions, especially Lyme disease and dengue fever, nearly every organ of the body can be affected to a greater or lesser extent, which is why the symptoms can be so variable, and the person can feel so ill. This variability is almost diagnostic of such conditions, especially as there are no satisfactory blood tests to prove the diagnosis. The reason for this is that there may be a number of different organisms involved, each having a different life cycle. In these cases it will take a little longer to achieve a resolution of the condition, as each organism is destroyed in its own time.

Years of "leeching" from dental amalgams can "innocently" deposit enough mercury in one's system to steal innocence, rob vitality, and erase precious memories. Lead can accumulate over the years from atmospheric exposure. Dislodging and vaporizing either or both of them may feel uncomfortable for a short time compared to the time it took for them to accumulate.

If there is nothing for chlorine dioxide to encounter, it deteriorates into constituents that are totally non-toxic. Nothing poisonous is left behind to build up, as is the case with many medical protocols. Medical treatments currently provide you no way of removing the poisons when they don't work. Chlorine dioxide, on the other hand, lasts long enough to do its job, and then the amount that does not furnish the immune system with needed ions becomes nothing more than micro amounts of salt and water. The chlorine dioxide has just a few minutes to do its job, and then it no longer exists, leaving nothing behind that can build up, or do additional harm.

The Procedure

The procedure for taking MMS is simple. All you need is your bottle of MMS, a clean, empty, dry glass, an eyedropper and the activator citric acid.

Note: When following the instructions below, keep this paragraph in mind. Always activate the MMS drops with one of the food acids, either lemon juice drops, or limejuice drops, or citric acid solution drops, the citric acid drops being the simplest.

Always add 5 drops of citric acid to each 1 drop of MMS, mix in an empty dry glass and wait at least 3 minutes, then add 1/3 to 2/3 glass of water and drink it. (You can expand the 3 minutes to 10 before drinking.)

Repeat this dose in between one and two hours, ideally doing all of this after your evening meal, possibly starting about ¾ hour after you have eaten, as it can sometimes make some people sleepy, apart from which your body does most of its detoxifying during the night.

Start modestly with as little as 1 drop of MMS plus 5 drops of citric acid on your first day (never forget to wait at least 3 minutes for the mixture to react to create chlorine dioxide, which will turn yellow and smell of chlorine, and repeat the dose in one to two hours). Take your time and do not rush. You could stay on this low dose for a few days, and then increase the number (2 and 10, 3 and 15, etc) on subsequent days, but I repeat – TAKE YOUR TIME. There is no point in going higher than 15 and 75 respectively, but it is rare for anyone to reach this level.

Your body will tell you when you've reached the optimum dosage for you, and, if in doubt, drop the next dose. Clearing may be a bit uncomfortable, but it need not be intolerable. You may feel like you've been through a battle, and, in a sense, you have. However I suggest that, if you develop any symptoms of any sort, assume you have taken too high a dose, so put up with the effect, take the antidote, and drop the next dose, possibly even not taking any for a day.

Before you can be healthy again, you need to destroy toxins, pathogens, parasites and anything harmful to you. In order to do so, they have to be uprooted and released from their "strongholds" in your body tissue. You have no idea what they are or where they are. Remember they may be buried deep in your organs.

You don't have to reach your maximum tolerated dose. Whatever dose you use will have its value, but the higher you can comfortably reach the better. It is just that the whole process will take that much longer.

This gentle approach applies to any chronic condition, and especially if you want to clean up your body. However, if you develop an acute medical condition such as dengue fever or malaria, for example, start straight in at at least 5 drops of MMS to 25 drops of citric acid, although you could possibly start at 8 drops of MMS to 40 drops of citric acid, and don't forget to repeat the dose in between one and two hours.

With any luck you will feel remarkably better by the next day. If you are not quite symptom free, repeat the same the next day, increasing the dose by about one third. In an acute situation, you can take three doses a day, each one repeated one to two hours later.

Antidote. If you develop any symptoms you don't like, assume it is the chlorine dioxide working too hard within you. To clear these symptoms, either take a few doses of ½ teaspoonful of sodium bicarbonate in a glass of water or a few grammes of vitamin C in water. Don't take both. Then either don't take a dose of MMS for 24 hours or drop the next dose and gradually work back up again.

IMPORTANT. Please be aware that, as I have already said, chlorine dioxide is a very potent chemical and literally destroys anything potentially harmful it comes across. Whatever dose you take, it will do its job. It is understandable that you want to reach as high a dose as possible as soon as possible, but I would encourage you not to think like that. As most of us have accumulated a lot of undesirable things within our bodies over the years, some of which may now be causing a major illness, it is not unreasonable to suggest that it may take some time to get rid of it all, possibly six months or more.

A number of people have reported to me that they did not feel any nausea, nor did they vomit, but started to feel generally unwell, or some of their old symptoms started to come back a bit, when they had reached a certain dose of chlorine dioxide. Fortunately they rang me. My advice was that they should go back to a lower dose, possible even not taking any chlorine dioxide for 24 hours before restarting at the lower dose. This approach has worked in every case. Unlike an antibiotic, nothing can develop a resistance to chlorine dioxide, as has already been said.

So what I am really trying to say is that, if you have ANY undesirable effects, even if you become a bit more tired than before, ASSUME that the chlorine dioxide is being too active for your body's current ability to eliminate the toxins. Take a lower dose next time, and be prepared to stay low for a while. Please don't overdose. It will only make you feel unnecessarily ill.

Overall you may feel the effects, but this is a good thing. You will also feel healthy again. Any sick feeling will be TEMPORARY, a small price to pay for the longer-term possibility of lasting restored health, no matter what stage of life you happen to be currently experiencing. When the clearing is done, you won't need to take the maximum dose. You can go on a maintenance application (1 or 2 drops of MMS) to keep your insides pathogen free and your immune system strong or take a dose every so often. I hope you have found this information helpful. In summary, when MMS is combined with citric acid it produces chlorine dioxide, which, at the appropriate dose is a safe and effective way to boost your immune system and eliminate a full range of harmful organisms, toxic metals and chemicals which may well be making you ill.

Dr. Patrick Kingsley. February 2008.

Next, while we are on the topic of simple chemical substances, let's look at two others: first, hydrogen peroxide...

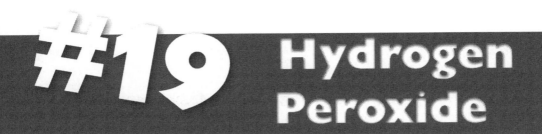

#19 Hydrogen Peroxide

The bleach story continues!
Hydrogen Peroxide: A Powerful Antibiotic

Hydrogen peroxide is like water (H_2O) with an extra oxygen atom added (H_2O_2). It's the extra oxygen and the power to release it right in the tissues that makes this substance a powerful medicine. Oxygen is good for us and bad for a great many pathogens, notably anaerobic bacteria, yeasts and viruses. It also cripples cancer cells and renders them vulnerable to the immune system.

Nature supplies us with abundant hydrogen peroxide. Every time it rains, falling drops of water bring down ozone from higher in the atmosphere in the form of hydrogen peroxide. The extra life-giving oxygen is undoubtedly one of the reasons plants do better when watered from the sky than from a watering can. It is also why rain is so refreshing. Don't hide indoors! Go out and get the extra oxygen: it's Nature's gift of energy!

In fact hydrogen peroxide from the sky is so good that farmers are known to mimic it by spraying their crops with diluted hydrogen peroxide. Feed it to your plants, using one ounce of 3% hydrogen peroxide solution to a quart of water. They'll love it!

Unfortunately, because of current atmospheric pollution, much of the peroxide never reaches the ground. It gets used up interacting with chemicals in the atmosphere and in urban areas this has lowered oxygen levels from the 20% you were taught in school, down to as little as 10%.

Despite its health-giving properties, our oxygen needs are not being met. The oxygen-generating rain forests are being destroyed worldwide, which further reduces available oxygen. Chlorination of drinking water removes oxygen. Cooking and over-processing of our foods lowers their oxygen content. Unrestrained antibiotic use destroys beneficial oxygen-creating bacteria in the intestinal tract.

Dr. Johanna Budwig of Germany has shown that for proper cellular utilization of oxygen to take place, our diets must contain adequate amounts of unsaturated fatty acids, rich in pi electrons. Unfortunately, the oils rich in these fatty acids have become less and less popular with the food industry. Their very reactive nature means they require more careful processing and it gives them a shorter shelf-life. The food industry, which has no apparent interest in human health, has therefore turned to the use of synthetic fats and dangerous processes like hydrogenation.

A Bit Of Biochemistry

Ozone is an unstable coupling of 3 oxygen atoms and it easily gives up the third oxygen atom which, once alone, becomes a violent reactor and can cause damage. That's why ozone is potentially hazardous. Hydrogen peroxide also has an extra oxygen atom, which it gives up easily, reverting to water. It too is potentially dangerous—but only if you misuse and abuse it, which of course is true of any medicine!

The fiery "singlet oxygen", as it's called, that is given up in the tissues is what creates the powerful medicinal properties of hydrogen peroxide. It's deadly to pathogens and deadly to cancer cells, yet does our bodies little harm.

The bubbling you see when hydrogen peroxide comes in contact with a bacteria-laden cut or wound is the oxygen being released and bacteria being destroyed.

You've probably understood the anti-oxidant story and you no doubt take antioxidants to protect yourself. However the missing half of the story, which rarely gets told by half-educated health "experts", is that we need oxygenation in our bodies. Hydrogen peroxide is the exact substance by which our own white blood cells kill bacteria, molds (yeasts) and viruses. Cells release it on the spot and then rapidly re-absorb and neutralize it when it has killed the pathogen.

If this ability was totally swamped by excessive anti-oxidants, then we wouldn't be able to fight off infections. Please remember this point. The ability of our cells to produce hydrogen peroxide is essential for life. H_2O_2 is not some undesirable by-product or toxin as orthodox medicine would have you believe, but instead a basic requirement for good health.

Hydrogen peroxide is involved in many other important processes in the body. For example, vitamin C helps fight infections by enhancing hydrogen peroxide production, which in turn stimulates the production of prostaglandins. Also lactobacillus found in the colon and vagina produce hydrogen peroxide. This destroys harmful bacteria and viruses, preventing colon disease, vaginitis, bladder infections and a host of other common ailments *(Infect Dis News Aug.8,91:5)*. It is required for the production of thyroid hormone and sexual hormones. *(Mol Cell Endocrinol 86;46(2): 149-154) (Steroids 82;40(5):5690579)*. It stimulates the production of interferon *(J Immunol 85;134(4):24492455)*. It dilates blood vessels in the heart and brain *(Am J Physiol 86;250 (5 pt 2): H815-821 and (2 pt 2):H157-162)*. It may improve glucose utilization in diabetics *(Proceedings of the IBOM Conference 1989, 1990, 1991)*.

The good thing is that hydrogen peroxide is dirt cheap and readily available. BUT YOU MUST TAKE CARE TO USE ONLY THE CORRECT FOOD GRADE FORM. More about that later.

We don't yet fully understand the complete workings of hydrogen peroxide but we do know that it is a prolific source of free oxygen. 1 pint of food-grade (35% solution) contains the equivalent of 130 pints of oxygen. 1 pint of 3% hydrogen peroxide found at the local drugstore contains 10 pints of oxygen. And 1 pint of the 6% solution (the kind used to bleach hair) contains 20 pints of oxygen.

We also know that when H_2O_2 is taken into the body (orally or intravenously) the oxygen content of the blood and body tissues increases dramatically. Early researchers felt these increases were simply due to the extra oxygen molecule being released. This is unlikely. Only very diluted amounts of H202 are ever introduced into the body. The small amount of oxygen present couldn't be solely responsible for the dramatic changes that take place.

Dr. Charles Farr, a strong proponent of intravenous use, has suggested another possible answer. He believes that hydrogen peroxide stimulates enzyme systems throughout the body. This triggers an increase in the metabolic rate, causes small arteries to dilate and increase blood flow, enhances the body's distribution and consumption of oxygen and raises body temperature *(Proceedings of the International Conference on Bio-Oxidative Medicine 1989, 1990, 1991)*.

A Little History

The therapeutic benefits of hydrogen peroxide were reported as far back as 1920. The prestigious English medical journal, The Lancet, carried the story that IV hydrogen peroxide was used to successfully treat pneumonia in the flu epidemic following World War I.

In the 1940's Father Richard Willhelm, a pioneer in promoting peroxide use, reported its extensive use in treating everything from bacterial-related mental illness to skin disease and polio. Father Willhelm founded of "Educational Concern for Hydrogen Peroxide" (ECHO, a nonprofit organization dedicated to educating the public on the safe use and therapeutic benefits of hydrogen peroxide).

Much of the interest in hydrogen peroxide waned in the 1940's when prescription medications came on the scene. Since that time there has been little economic interest in funding peroxide research. After all, it is inexpensive and non-patentable, so worthless to drug companies, who pursue profits above patient care. Yet despite this lack of apparent interest of orthodox medicine, over 7,700 articles relating to hydrogen peroxide have been written in the standard medical journals.

Thousands more, involving its therapeutic use, have appeared in alternative health publications. The number of conditions helped by hydrogen peroxide is astounding. The reported dangers and side effects are few and often conflicting.

Again, I repeat, that it is quite safe if handled properly. But deadly if not.

Only 35% Food Grade hydrogen peroxide is recommended for internal use. See overleaf for notes about grades of hydrogen peroxide.

Even at this concentration, however, hydrogen peroxide is a very strong oxidizer and if not diluted, it can be extremely dangerous or even fatal. Any concentrations over 10% can cause neurological reactions and damage to the upper gastrointestinal tract. There have been two known fatalities in children who ingested 27% and 40% concentrations of H202.

Recently, a 26 month old female swallowed one mouthful of 35% H202. She immediately began vomiting, followed by fainting and respiratory arrest. Fortunately, she was soon under emergency room care and although she experienced erosion and bleeding of the stomach and esophagus, she survived the incident. When she was re-examined 12 days later, the areas involved had healed *(J Toxicol Clin Toxicol 90;28(1):95-100)*.

What Diseases Can Be Treated With Hydrogen Peroxide?

All infections will benefit, whether viral, bacterial, fungal (yeasts and molds) or parasitic. The list would be long but would include colds, influenza, Herpes, sore throats, gum (periodontal) disease, infected wounds and burns, MRSA certainly, pneumonia, hepatitis, infectious mononeucleosis, Lyme, vaginal Thrush, bowel disorders (proctitis, colitis, Crohn's etc), prostatitis, trichomoniasis, systemic Candiasis and cystitis.

Veterinary parasitology also suggests it is effective against toxoplamosis, which is otherwise almost impossible to treat *[Veterinary Parasitology, Volume 153, Issues 3-4, 31 May 2008, s 209-213]*.

Even claims have been made for the successful treatment of AIDS (these are never investigated for their worth; the doctors are just treated as liars and quacks).

How Is Peroxide Used?

In serious situations and if local political matters permit, there is no question that hydrogen peroxide (and ozone) therapies are best administered by a qualified health professional, who know what he or she is doing.

But you can do it for yourself, if you can get the correct grade of hydrogen peroxide. For the avoidance of confusion, here is information about all the common forms of hydrogen peroxide. Be sure you understand what you are buying, if you want to use it for self-therapy.

Grades of Hydrogen Peroxide

Hydrogen peroxide is available in various strengths and grades.

1. 90%: This is used as an oxygen source for rocket fuel!

2. 3.5% Pharmaceutical Grade: This is the grade sold at your local drugstore or supermarket. This product is not recommended for internal use. It contains an assortment of stabilizers which shouldn't be ingested. Various

stabilizers include: acetanilide, phenol, sodium stanate and tertrasodium phosphate.

3. 6% Beautician Grade: This is used in beauty shops to color hair and is not recommended for internal use.

4. 30% Reagent Grade: This is used for various scientific experimentation and also contains stabilizers. It is also not for internal use.

5. 30% to 32% Electronic Grade: This is used to clean electronic parts and not for internal use.

6. 35% Technical Grade: This is a more concentrated product than the Reagent Grade and differs slightly in that phosphorus is added to help neutralize any chlorine from the water used to dilute it.

7. 35% Food Grade: This is used in the production of foods like cheese, eggs, and whey-containing products. It is also sprayed on the foil lining of aseptic packages containing fruit juices and milk products. Only 35% Food Grade hydrogen peroxide is recommended for internal use. At this concentration, however, hydrogen peroxide is a very strong oxidizer and if not diluted, it can be extremely dangerous or even fatal.

You must handle it without getting it on your skin. Direct contact will burn the skin. Rubber gloves from Home Depot or similar are recommended. If you do get any on your skin, wash it off immediately with copious water.

It needs to be diluted down to 3%. Diluting 10 times would result in 3.5%, so if we dilute it 1 in 12, that's close to 3%. You can do this easily by pouring 1 ounce of H2O2 into a pint jug or jar, then adding 11 ounces of distilled water. This will make 12 ounces of 3%.

I recommend that you transfer the H_2O_2 as you need it to a small glass eyedropper bottle, which you can get from your local drugstore. Leave the rest in the tightly sealed bottle it came in and store it at the back of the refrigerator, where it will be quite stable chemically, for long periods (make sure children cannot access it).

Suggested Dose Regime

Based on years of experience and thousands of cases reports, the following dose regime is known to work well and should be right for you.

Drops can be added to 6- 8 ounces of liquid in a glass, either more distilled water, fruit juice, milk or aloe vera (juice or gel). DO NOT USE TAP WATER: the chlorine in tapwater would deactivate the hydrogen peroxide.

Hydrogen peroxide must be taken only on an empty stomach. If there is food in the stomach, the reaction on any bacteria present may cause excess foaming, indigestion, and possibly even vomiting. Additionally, some animal research indicates that when it is given orally, peroxide combines with iron and small amounts of vitamin C in the stomach, hydroxyl radicals are created *(J Inorg Biochem 89;35(1):55-69).*

Day	Number of Drops	Time Per Day
1	3	3
2	4	3
3	5	3
4	6	3
5	7	3
6	8	3
7	9	3
8	10	3
9	12	3
10	14	3
11	16	3
12	18	3
13	20	3
14	22	3
15	24	3
16	25	3

Please don't go above 25 drops. It may be counter-productive.

Transplant patients should not take hydrogen peroxide. It strongly stimulates the immune system and could, theoretically, cause a rejection of the organ. If you feel nauseated and sick, this could be a healing crisis. As you detox and kill off lots of pathogens in your system, your body may not be able to remove the breakdown products fast enough. The answer is just to persist until the toxins are cleared.

Try to keep going at the dose you are on; just don't increase it until the reaction wears off. Then resume the climbing dose (maximum, 25 drops, 3 times a day).

You should also take vitamin E (alpha and gamma mixed forms, not synthetic alpha-tocopherol). It enhances oxygen metabolism and is quite safe, whatever the current scientific frenzy to discredit it.

You should also actively engage in pre- and probiotics (section #40a), to start repopulating your body with good friendly bacteria.

You can get food grade 35% hydrogen peroxide online at this website:

http://www.dfwx.com/h2o2.htm

Other Administration Routes For Hydrogen Peroxide

1. Three tablespoons mixed with a quart of distilled (or any non-chlorinated) water makes a good vaginal douche, for those stricken with bacterial or yeast (Candida) vaginitis.

   Remember the need to re-populate with good flora. The pH of the vagina is important.

   It is normally kept slightly low by malic acid. This deters bacteria and yeasts. I have heard (but don't recommend) women douching with yoghurt to increase friendly flora.

   One case was found with a raspberry seed stuck in her cervix: she'd used supermarket sweetened fruit yoghurt, which was very silly!

   Enemas. The above formula can also be used effectively for colon infection (Candida, Giardia and other).

2. It makes an effective full strength mouthwash or can be mixed with baking soda for toothpaste.

3. It can be used full strength as a foot bath for athlete's foot. (Diabetics have found relief from circulation problems by soaking their feet in 1 pint of 3% peroxide mixed with 1 gallon of warm, non-chlorinated water for 30 minutes nightly.)

4. A tablespoon added to 1 cup of non-chlorinated water can be used as a nasal spray. Depending on the degree of sinus involvement, one will have to adjust the amount of peroxide used. If it causes excess catarrhal discharge, reduce the proportions.

#20 Hydrochloric acid Injections

What? That's right. Only 1:1,000 strength! It's more barefoot doctoring from the days before fancy antibiotics. Burr Ferguson M.D. of Birmingham AL first wrote about it around 1925. Dr. Ferguson had been a battle surgeon during World War 1 and he had seen the wounded die by the hundreds from infections. He quickly found that when 10 mls of 1:1,000 hydrochloric acid is given IV, there is a rapid and significant increase in the white cell count. Infections melted away and fever subsided.

You can treat virtually any infection with this simple protocol. It's quite safe!

Begin as soon as there are signs of fever. Shots are given daily. Usually after a week the fever is cleared and the patient feeling well.

The doctor was William Howell M.D. of Lexington, Tennessee told of the following case in a 1930s journal Medical World:

The patient was age 15 and she was delivered of a very large baby that lived only for two hours. She lived in a log cabin in the woods. The delivery was done with the best aseptic condition that could be had in a log cabin. The patient weighed only 90 pounds. There were some small lacerations. On day three after delivery there was a message that the patient had a chill and high fever. She lived in a river bottom and I was in hope that it was malaria and I sent quinine. On the fifth day there was another message telling of the grave condition of the patient. In going into the sick room I saw at once that the message had been urgent. The girl was delirious, temperature was 106, pulse was 140, respiration was 40 and there was a discharge from the vagina with a fetid odor. Every other case I had seen like her had died of the infection.

I had some one in 1,500 hydrochloric acid with me but had feared to use it. I injected 10 cc of 1 in 1,500 hydrochloric acid into a vein with much trepidation. The following minutes were anxious ones for me as I hardly knew what to expect. I had never heard of hydrochloric acid being used to treat puerperal sepsis. I was thinking of the warnings of the fatal results of an injection of acid in the vein. I was holding the radial pulse when all of a sudden there was sweat on the patient's neck and forehead and a slowing of the pulse. In a few more minutes the patient was bathed in a profuse perspiration and there was a stop to the chatter of her delirium. Thirty minutes after the injection she was conscious and I asked her how she felt. She said that she felt much better. She wanted to go to sleep.

Within an hour of the injection, her temperature had dropped to 103, her pulse had dropped to 100 and respiration had decreased to 22. On the next four days I repeated the injections. On day six, temperature was 99, pulse was 72 and respiration was 19. Two days later I was called and told that her fever had returned. Her temperature was 101 and there was a free discharge from the vagina. I gave her one more injection of 10 cc of acid.

All signs of the infection she had had completely disappeared.

The story was later retold by Barry Groves in Townsend Letter for Doctors, December 2001 issue.

Obviously this is one remedy that should probably only be done by an MD or RN. But in an emergency, in the jungle, anywhere, just do it!

I've administered hydrochloric acid to myself IV on two occasions. It worked and was entirely without side effects. If you end up with MRSA or any other dangerous or intractable infection, don't trust to antibiotics to save you: get some holistic practitioner to do this protocol for you.

I need hardly say that I believe it would be wise for decent MDs to re-learn these older techniques which certainly worked. Moreover they were cheap and safe (that was partly the problem, of course: no major drug company would ever promote such profit-less remedies).

One more case from Dr. William Howell, then we're done:

The acid gives the same happy results in nephritis. Give an injection every day---in five or six days the albumin diminishes until there is none. I saw a case of acute nephritis September, 1933, following scarlet fever. A boy, nine years of age, swollen till he looked as though he would burst. I tried everything I could get at; salt-free diet, potassium citrate in large doses, milk diet. The hospital authorities said his urine showed four plus albumin. After six weeks he showed no improvement.

I decided to try the acid. I gave him 3 c.c. of a 1:500 solution in the gluteal muscle every day, alternating hips each day. In seven days the albumin began to decrease. After twenty-one injections he was entirely well. I have reports from him almost weekly; no albumin.

I saw him May 6th, 1934. He was out on the road with other children, was just as busy in their games as they were, showed no signs of his former trouble, looked well, ruddy like the others. Since that time I saw another case of acute prostatitis, urine loaded with albumin. After six injections his urine was entirely cleared up. I have given him about twenty-five injections. He sleeps well at night; no more bladder trouble.

I have a man under my care who had tuberculosis of the lungs. The bladder became involved. I gave him an injection every day for thirty days. He missed his fever, all bladder symptoms are gone, eats plenty, sleeps well, has had no fever in ten months. His weight has gone up from 140 to 180 lbs. I am still giving him an injection once a week. He is doing light work, coughs very little. He has taken more than one hundred injections with never the slightest harm.

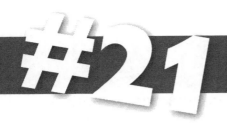

If you've been into alternative and holistic medicine for any length of time. You must have heard of colloidal silver is an anti-septic. You've probably heard that Alexander the Great's troops kept their water supply in silver vessels and how wagon train pioneers, travelling through the Wild West, used to put a silver dollar in the water barrel, to keep the water pure.

There is really no argument that it is effective. In fact, silver has even reached the mainstream in the form of silver-soaked bandage line from Curad. According to the bandage company: "Laboratory testing showed that silver reduced bacterial growth like Staph. aureus, E. coli, E. hirae and Pseudomonas aeruginosa -- a powerful germ that does not respond to many antibacterials -- in the dressing for 24 hours."

Even washing machines are now, for better or worse, using silver ions to kill bacteria.

Meanwhile, silver-coated urinary catheters are used to help reduce urinary tract infections (UTIs) -- studies showed they reduced the incidence of UTI by 47 percent.

Silver inhibits the growth of bacteria by deactivating the bacteria's oxygen metabolism enzymes. In turn, this destroys the bacteria's cell membranes, stopping the replication of the bacteria's DNA. *[Source- Acupoll Precision Research, April 2003 Beiersdorf, Inc.]*

The real problem is not credibility with colloidal silver antisepsis. The problem is that there's an awful lot of junk products, manufactured in garage and kitchen top businesses, with small and inadequate electrolysis machines. These are really not potent enough to have any noticeable effect. Yet the people who peddle these goods like to quote science to give them credibility.

Don't be fooled, make sure you get a good product. It's not just a matter of the particle count but particle size also (surface area)—and ionic silver content.

Silver ions are silver atoms which have an electron missing in the outer shell. Silver particles are metallic silver consisting of clusters of silver atoms and can range in size from less than a nanometer up to 1,000 nanometers (1 micron). Silver ions will combine with chloride ions readily where they are present. The human stomach contains a strong solution of hydrochloric acid. Silver chloride forms immediately in the stomach when silver ions enter it. The same thing happens to silver ions in the bloodstream by virtue of the high chloride content due to the presence of sodium and potassium chloride. Silver ions, therefore are of little value inside the body as they are quickly combined with the available chloride ions to form worthless silver chloride.

Let me suggest a product called Advanced Colloidal Silver. It has approximately 20% ionic silver and 80% silver particles with a mean average of about 2 nanometers. This small particle size, combined with small particles results in a vastly larger surface area of silver for a given concentration. Because of this, ACS is potentially more effective than those products with much larger particles and much higher ppms.

The difference between good and bad products is illustrated by a study carried out by Dr. Ron Leavitt of BYU University, and reported by Deseret News, Tuesday, May 16, 2000.

According to Leavitt "The data suggests that with the low toxicity associated with colloidal silver, in general, and the broad spectrum of antimicrobial activity of this colloidal silver preparation, this preparation may be effectively used as an alternative to antibiotics."

The original study compared a good quality colloidal silver against tetracyclines, fluorinated quinolones (Ofloxacin), the penicillins, the cephalosporins (Cefaperazone) and the macrolides (Erythromycin). Among the microbes tested were streptococcuses, pneumonia, E. coli, salmonella, and shigella.

There has since been considerable dispute about Leavitt's right to publish this data publicly, with BYU sending intimidating cease and desist orders out to individuals and organizations referencing the study. These letters go beyond reasonable demand that copyrights be respected and further demand that BYU not be mentioned in conjunction with the study at all, despite the fact this information now exists in the public domain.

Safety Of Colloidal Silver

Up until the advent of chemical antibiotics which came about in the 1940's, some very strong silver products were being used as antibiotics. Of the millions of people who used these concentrated silver products, there were no reported deaths and only 239 reported cases of generalized Argyria (EPA Report ECAO-CIN-026 Jan "91" Pg. VI-3). In that same EPA report on VI-4 it states that Gaul and Staud (1935) suggested 8 grams of silver arsphenamine (used by injection at 145,000 ppm strength) as a safe total (lifetime) dose.

They also noted that other authors suggest safe total doses of 12-15 grams, based on clinical experience. The work of Furchner et al (1968) as stated above showed that small amounts of silver did not build up in the system of primates.

According to the EPA IRIS Report on silver (Integrated Risk Information Systems) (5th , 1st paragraph) it states that a number of tests were completed to investigate the absorption and retention of ingested silver in a number of animals (including primates). In conclusion, the test work indicated that between 90-99% of ingested silver was excreted on the second day after ingestion and greater than 99% was excreted in less than a week.

In other words, almost all the ingested silver was out of the body in only two days, which indicates that silver does not build up in the system when consumed in small amounts.

Overdose (Argyria)

However, it is possible to overdose with silver, and this may lead to a rare cosmetic condition of blue skin. Its scientific name is argyria or silverism and is an irreversible blue-gray discoloration of the skin, nails and gums that's linked to colloidal silver. It can happen gradually and sneak up on you unawares, after a number of years.

You have to be pretty excessive (in fact really daft) to get it. It would require an intake of 1,000 mgm or more from the use of any silver compound, including its salts. Once established, the condition is usually permanent and is a kind of disfigurement.

The US Federal Register listed the silver products that cause argyria as silver salts, including; silver nitrate, silver arsphenamine, silver chloride and possibly silver iodide. These products were sold until about 1975 under various labels consisting of silver solutions ranging from 5-30% silver [50,000-300,000 ppm (parts per million) of silver] *(Federal Register, FDA-21CFR Part 310, pg. 53685)*.

In comparison American Biotech Labs silver supplement products are only 10 ppm and 22 ppm. American Biotech Labs' EPA approved hospital/home surface disinfectant is only 32 ppm.

Other potential side effects of the liquid include: seizures and other neurological problems Kidney damage Indigestion Headaches and fatigue Skin irritation

Now let's look at nutritional factors against infections. It's CRITICAL!

I have already explained that the main reason TB was conquered had nothing to do with vaccines or antibiotics; it was just improvement in nutrition for the population. It's the same story for most infectious diseases. The usually touted nonsense that we've conquered disease with antibiotics and vaccinations is completely wrong but it's believed with all the passion of religious fervor, directly against all evidence to the contrary.

Here's the proof:

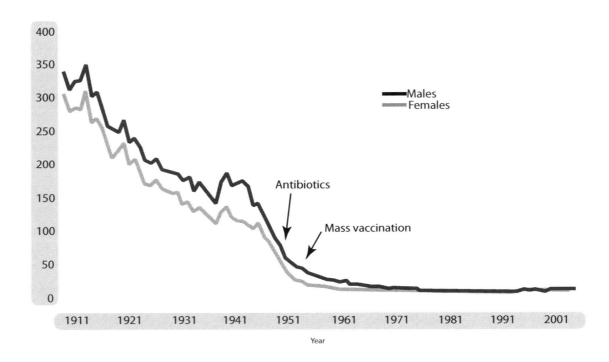

These figures are from Britain but the trend is the same the whole world over.

And TB (overleaf):

Note the sudden surge during the Second World War. This was due to temporary malnutrition and further re-inforces the point I am trying to make.

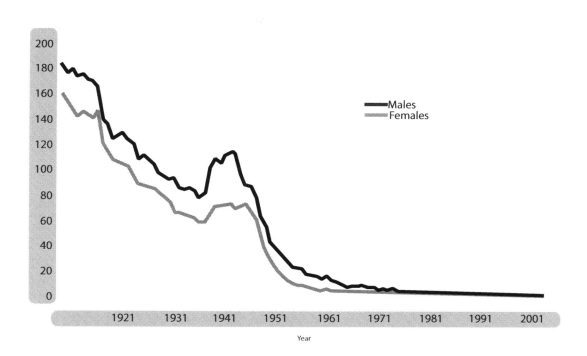

Year

This is typical of all the developed world, including the USA. For instance, from the years 1900 to 1945 (around the time penicillin started to become available) USA deaths from dipththeria declined from an average of 40 per 100,000 to just 2!

General standards of hygiene and wellbeing, good housing, plus adequate nutrition made a big difference in general immunity in the population.

Nutrition bullets

This is not a book on nutrition but here, in a nutshell, is what you should do.

Avoid sugar at all costs. You probably know that in the US the average per capita is 150 lbs. That's 3 lbs a week! Over 150 years ago Native American Indians warned against sugar: they said it weakened the body. It makes the immune system sluggish for up to 6 hours afterwards and the last thing you would want is tardy white blood cells that show up late for the action! Also it removes zinc which is very important for immunity.

Eat well. By that I mean a natural diet of natural foods with enough calories. Infectious diseases prosper only where there is malnutrition. Almost all endemic diseases (diseases which run permanently in society, not just in epidemic fashion), such as measles, TB and cholera, all declined significantly in the decades BEFORE antibiotics. The cause was better nutrition.

Remember being overweight does not mean you have "extra" nutrition: it means you have mal- or dys-nutrition. You are eating badly, eating the wrong things and ruining your body defences.

Alcohol, caffeine and tobacco are also known to lower immunity.

Instead of junk you must eat more foods containing anti-oxidants. These are contained in colored fruits, especially berries, blue, red and black. Manufactured foods which contain none of these essential life-giving food properties. It's astonishing how little infectious disease you will ever get, if you eat like this.

You will hear talk from some people who do not do their research properly that vitamin D is the "antibiotic vitamin". It is not. Vitamin A is the clear winner. For my subscribers to the Wholesome Living Letter (now ceased publication) I cited important clinical trials in the years before antibiotics that vitamin A in very large doses (50- 100,000 IU) killed virulent bacteria as well as antibiotics. Mortality rates moved from 100% fatal to 100% survival. That's BETTER than antibiotics!

In 1929 a milestone study was conducted by Sir Edward Mellanby, Professor of Pharmacology in Sheffield, England, for the Medical Research Council of the UK. Up to that time, puerperal sepsis was a highly fatal and untreatable condition (for instance in 1928, just one year earlier, there were 16 cases on Mellanby's pitch and all the women died). Mellanby administered high doses of vitamin A to 5 women in his study—one of the first controlled clinical trials ever—and all 5 women survived! It was a triumph for science but also nutrition.

Unfortunately, antibiotics lay just around the corner and that soon put paid to the idea of a humble vitamin being remarkably effective against a killer fever. Well, please remember, just 80 years on, the clock has turned completely and we are now almost post-antibiotics. *[Mellanby E, Green HE (1929). Vitamin A as an anti-infective agent. Its use in the treatment of puerperal septicaemia. BMJ 1:984-6]*

In 1931, Mellanby published another keynote paper with the title 'Diet as a prophylactic agent against puerperal sepsis'. In it he measured the incidence of 'sepsis' in a group of 550 post-natal women. Yet the list included cystitis (9 cases), mastitis (7 cases), influenza (1 case), gonorrhea (1 case), cervicitis (1 case) and septic perineum (2 cases), endometritis (7 cases) and 1 case of streptococcal septicaemia.

Again the response to Vitamin A was remarkable. [Green HN, Pindar D, Davis G, Mellanby E (1931). Diet as a prophylactic agent against puerperal sepsis, with special reference to Vitamin A as an anti-infective agent. BMJ 2:595-598].

What is meant by high doses of vitamin A? 25,000 – 50,000 units. "But that's toxic", say the pundits, aghast. Well, which would you choose: vitamin overdose or death? The fact is that vitamin A is not toxic at these levels in the short term. Your fate is decided in 48- 72 hours! Not long enough to worry about liver toxicity, surely?

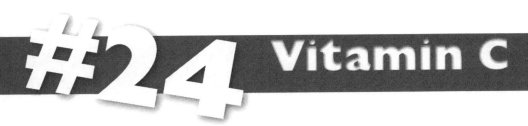

Now come to what is probably the most powerful of all antibiotic substances known to man. Incredibly, it's also one of the safest pharmaceuticals we have. If you are caught in a vicious pandemic, yet you can gain access to this therapy, you should do fine!

I'm talking about humble vitamin C (ascorbic acid). Actually not so humble—it has brought people out of septicemic coma when nothing else worked and regular antibiotics were powerless to save the patient.

But only when administered IV in huge doses, hundreds of times greater than doctors today would even consider.

The full story of its power is told in an important book, entitled Vitamin C Infectious Diseases And Toxins (Curing The Incurable) by Thomas E. Levy MD, JD. The author cites over 12,000 medical and scientific journal references, which is far more than I can do here.

Levy's book leans a great deal on the work of an earlier doctor called Frederick R. Klenner MD, chief of staff at the Memorial Hospital in Reidsville, North Carolina, who worked in the 30s and 40s, when vitamin C first became readily available as an affordable pharmaceutical.

Klenner pioneered his treatment on hundreds of cases and had outstanding results against many infectious diseases, using intravenous vitamin C.

Klenner maintained hospital records and fever charts that told of case after case of recovery from meningitis, encephalitis, pneumonia and serious complications following scarlet fever (Streptococcus). Many fevers from 100-105 degrees F began to diminish within minutes of intravenous vitamin C. Both viral and bacterial diseases responded. The only requirement seemed to be that the dose was large enough and treatment continued for long enough.

Polio Teasers

Adelle Davies, famous authoress of the classic text Let's Eat Right to Keep Fit, was fortunate enough to meet Dr Klenner, and she tells us one of his stories; of an 18-month-old girl suffering from polio. The mother reported that the child had become paralysed following a convulsion, after which she soon lost consciousness. When Dr Klenner first saw the child her little body was blue, stiff, and cold to the touch; he could neither hear heart sounds nor feel a pulse; her rectal temperature was 100°F. The only sign of life, he could detect was a suggestion of moisture condensed on a mirror held to her mouth. The distraught mother was convinced that the child was already dead.

Klenner injected 6000 mg of vitamin C into the child's blood; four hours later she was cheerful and alert, holding a bottle with her right hand, though her left hand was still paralysed.

A second injection was given; soon the child was laughing and holding her bottle with both hands, all signs of paralysis gone. She recovered fully.

To show just how far this can be pushed, Levy cites an adult case, a woman, also a polio victim. She had considerable pain in the hamstring area, pain in neck and pain in the lower back. She had a natural desire to keep her entire body static to avoid painful movements. Her fever reached 104.6°F, along with a sore throat that had relapsed after initial treatment with antibiotics, aspirin and fruit juice two weeks earlier.

Although the patient weighed less than 120 lbs. Klenner nevertheless immediately administered 22,000 mg (22 g) of vitamin C. by slow intravenous injection, using a large 100 cc syringe. Plus he prescribed 1500 mg of vitamin C with juice every two hours by mouth.

Twelve hours later, the woman was free of her headache, and her fever was down to 101.4°F. Klenner gave her another 22,000 mg injection; this caused nausea and vomiting which lasted for around 30 minutes. Then, 24 hours later, her temperature had further dropped to 100.8°F, with a definite clinical improvement.

She was continued on 18,000 mg injections given every 12 hours (equivalent to 36 g a day). After a few days, the IV vitamin C. was discontinued, but the patient was asked to continue by mouth for an additional week taking 1500 mg every three to four hour.

Klenner noted that the patient had an almost complete elimination of pain, except at the knees, after the first 48 hours. The temperature normalised in 84 hours. The patient finally made a complete recovery.

Although these are viral cases, similar outstanding results are to be obtained with potentially fatal bacterial infections, such as tetanus, diphtheria, pneumococcal pneumonia, TB, leprosy and typhoid fever. Klenner came to speak of vitamin C as "the antibiotic par excellence".

Blood Levels

Significantly, Klenner found that vitamin C levels vanished completely from the blood when the patient was under the stress of an acute infection. Nor could any vitamin C be found in the urine. This severe deficiency might be why patients respond so dramatically to massive doses of the vitamin. We now know that this lack is caused by vitamin C being used up by neutralizing toxins and blasting viruses and bacteria; it effectively eliminates the danger, but is lost in doing so.

The rational basis of the high dose technique is therefore to administer vitamin C intravenously until it began to spill over into the urine and could be detected once again. Monitoring blood levels is obviously even more accurate but not always possible and not necessarily desirable when urgency can save a life; after all, vitamin C is pretty harmless. In any case, it is the intracellular levels that count, which may be much depleted, even when blood plasma levels appear reasonable.

Hence Klenner's urgency and the need to administer the doses as rapidly as possible, to be sure the plasma was overloaded and thus that the vitamin C would be sure to flood into the cells. Modern research, by the way, shows us that white blood cells may carry up to 80 times the residual blood levels of vitamin C, thus being sure to bring plenty of it to the site of an infection. So Nature knows how good this stuff is!

Klenner published at least 20 significant papers and in 1949 addressed the American Medical Association, to tell colleagues what he'd achieved. Yet his work is now virtually lost and any mention of it is dismissed as myth and nonsense. The truth is now known only to a few physicians and practitioners [it was my "drug of choice' to take with me to the danger zone rescue mission after the 2004 tsunami and kindly donated by friend of Deseret Biologicals, Sandy, Utah].

Klenner achieved outstanding recoveries in diseases which at that time were considered to be virtually untreatable.

Bacterial Diseases

Thomas Levy also quotes extensive research by other scientists and doctors, using large doses of vitamin C to overcome severe and sometimes fatal bacterial infections, including the following:

- Rocky Mountain spotted fever.

- Pseudomonas, a notoriously difficult to treat bacteria.

- Bacillary dysentery and even amoebic dysentery.

- Brucellosis.

- Malaria (not a bacterial disease, but transmissible parasite called Plasmodium).

- Typhoid fever (not to be confused with typhus, which also responds but is viral in origin)

- Leprosy

- Staphylococcus

- Streptococcus (leads to rheumatic fever).

- Tuberculosis

- Tetanus,

- Whooping Cough (Pertussis)

- Diphtheria

Note also: studies have proven that large doses of vitamin C helps to prevent allergies of varying kinds. I've given IV gallons of the stuff over the years. It even counters the effects of poison oak, poison ivy, snakebite, black widow spider bite and carbon monoxide poisoning.

So if treatment with intravenous vitamin C is so effective in such a wide variety of conditions, how is it that most doctors have never even heard of it, much less use it in their office?

Klenner Protocol

The trouble is that the scientific literature is dogged with studies which purport to investigate the effects of vitamin C but which used such tiny doses as to be worthless. It is an almost universal mistake among doctors to believe that ascorbic acid has only vitamin like properties and these manifested only a few hundred milligrams at most. It is even cited in the literature that the body will block blood levels above about 300 mgms. What Thomas Levy turns to calling "Klenner-sized doses" of vitamin C are very large—around 500- 700 mgms per kg of body weight, repeated several times a day. That would range from 20 grams daily for an infant; 40 grams for a child; to 25 grams for a slight-built woman; to 50 grams for a hefty man.

Clearly this is beyond the vitamin nature of ascorbic acid and indicates that it has a very important detoxing and antimicrobial property.

This is critically important because most bacteria exert their deadly effect by means of a toxin. So a substance which both destroys the pathogens and their toxins is indeed a godsend.

Take diphtheria, which once had a dreadful mortality rate of 80% (now down to 5- 10%). This disease kills by the secretion of a sticky dense membrane, which forms in the throat and suffocates the child. But there is also a deadly toxin, Diphtheria A, which itself is rapidly fatal once present in sufficient quantity.

To treat this condition, Klenner recommended huge doses, as described, of 500- 700 mgm per kilogram of bodyweight, run into a vein through a wide bore needle "as fast as the cardiovascular system would allow". This is several thousand times what most doctors (in their ignorance) would consider safe. Yet even in these very high doses, ascorbic acid shows no ill effects on the patient, making vitamin C one of the most remarkable substances in human physiology.

There have been many published studies on this topic but in one report Klenner describes the fate of three children living in the same neighborhood, each with diphtheria. All three children had different doctors. The little girl under Klenner's scare was given 10 g of vitamin C in an intravenous push with a 50 cc syringe, every eight hours for the first 24 hours and then every 12 hours. She was also given 40,000 units of diphtheria antitoxin, injected into her abdomen. The other two children received the antitoxin as well, but they did not receive any vitamin C. They both died but Klenner's patient survived, later becoming a nurse.

[Klenner F. Observations of the dose and administration of ascorbic acid, when employed there are in the range of the vitamin in human pathology Journal Of Applied Nutrition, 23 (3&4); 61-88.]

It should be noted that Klenner's work with diphtheria is ably supported by other studies of the time. Harde and Philippe, demonstrated that lethal doses of diphtheria toxin premixed with vitamin C were no longer lethal when injected into guinea pigs. Without the vitamin C, the toxin killed the guinea pigs in just a few days. *[Harde E and Phillippe M. Observations sur le pouvoir antigene mélange toxine diphtherique et vitamin C. Compt rende Acad d sc 9:738-739]*

Levy cites several other studies from different countries, also showing vitamin C protected guinea pigs from the fatal effects of diphtheria toxin.

Streptococci and Staphylococci

What about these common human pathogens, which can produce infections varying from minor suffering to a fatal outcome? After all, we are very interested in Staph, because of MRSA.

Same great story. Vitamin C triumphs.

One study looked at two children with defective abilities of their white blood cells to kill bacteria. They are especially susceptible to repeated skin infections with staphylococcus. The study reported that vitamin C. was effective in delaying and eventually suppressing infectious episodes. *[Rebora A. and Crovato F. F Dallegri, and F. Patrone (1980) Repeated staphylococcal pyoderma in two siblings with defective neutraphil bacteria killing. Dermatologica 160(2):106-112].*

A much earlier study (1941) was able to demonstrate an inhibition of the growth of Staphylococcus aureus, even at relatively low doses. *[Gupta G. and B. Guha (1941) The effect of vitamin C and certain other substances on the growth of microorganisms. Annals of Biochemistry and Experimental Medicine 1(1):14-26]*

Kodama and Kojima were able to demonstrate the ability of vitamin C. to render staphylococcus related toxin, harmless. (Remember, I explained that the main deadly effect of virulent bacteria is the toxins that they produce). *[Kodama T. and T. Kojima (1939) Studies of the staphylococcal toxin, toxoid and antitoxin; effect of ascorbic acid and staphylococcal lysins and organsisms. Kitasato Archives of Experimental Medicine 16:36-55].*

Yet another case report described an elderly woman with an ulcer on her left cheek infected with the presence of staphylococcus aureus. She had had the condition over three years, but it rapidly healed with vitamin C therapy. *[Lederman E. (1962) Vitamin C deficiency and ulceration of the face. The Lancet 2:1382].*

Nakashini reported that the direct (topical) application of vitamin C to a bedsore was able to remarkably enhance the bacteria killing effect of antibiotics. He also noted that MRSA subsequently disappeared from the wound. *[Nakanishi T. (1992) [A report on a clinical experience of which has successfully made several antibiotic-resistant bacteria (MRSA etc) negative on a bedsore] Article in Japanese. Igaku Kenkyu. Acta Medica. 62(1):31-37.*

It even works in animals, test-tube experiments showed that the presence of vitamin C. significantly increase the ability of white blood cells to kill staphylococcus aureus.

[Andreason C. and Frank D. (1999) The effects of ascorbic acid on in vitro heterophil function. Avian Diseases 43(4):656-663.]

Remember the work I already alluded to, by Kelly (1944), showing that pathogens are almost universal in the mouths and on the tonsils of healthy hosts. It is only when immunity is compromised by nutritional deficiency— in this case lack of vitamin C—that infections can become established and overcome the host.

So in a way we are going round in circles and saying that good nutrition is your best protection against pathogens. If you do it right you may never even contract a disease, never mind succumb to it, even during a worldwide pandemic in which others are dying by the million!

But if you get MRSA, epidemic or not, make sure you call this section to the attention of a competent practitioner who is licensed to carry out this procedure. You will survive.

Administration

You will gather from reading this far that intravenous vitamin C can be a lifesaver, even for a patient afflicted with the most deadly infection and almost at the point of death.

But obviously not everyone will be able to find the help of a physician to administer IV vitamin C, especially in the event of a worldwide pandemic. To administer therapeutic doses to yourself, you only need to take vitamin C powder using the "fill and flush" method; that means to take doses by mouth, increasing by a teaspoonful at a time, until it causes diarrhea. We believe this happens only when the tissues have become saturated with the vitamin.

For a child, Adelle Davis suggests putting one cup of hot water in a liquifier, adding 50 tablets of vitamin C (500 mg each), blending well, sweeten to taste with honey, pour into a glass jar, and keep refrigerated. Doses can be administered mouthful at a time, or teaspoonful at that time.

If one does not have a liquifier, Davis suggest crushing 50 tablets and dissolving these in a cup of hot water. Each teaspoon of such a solution contains 500 mg. If 100 tablets (500 mg each) are dissolved in a cup of water, each teaspoon a solution would supply 1 g (1000 mg).

For any infectious disease in a sick child, mild or severe, administering a teaspoon more of vitamin C solution, sweetened in this way, can be a godsend when a physician cannot be reached, as for example, during the night.

Note that synthetic vitamin C does not contain enzymes found in natural foods; therefore it is quite stable to heat and storage. But once stirred into foods, such as fruit juice, enzymes will begin to activate and readily destroy it.

[Davies without any and L. let's eat right to keep fit, Harcourt Brace Jankovich, New York, 1954, 1970, 132 to 134]

There are no right and wrong doses of vitamin C as such. All these treatments are based on empirical experience (basically trial and error). But this wonderful natural substance is very tolerant of error, and it's almost impossible to overdose a person on it.

Vitamin C vs. Ascorbic Acid

Don't listen to the ignorant nonsense widespread on the Web that vitamin C is "good" and "natural", while ascorbic acid is "bad" and synthetic. They are both IDENTICAL in physiological properties; just different names for the same thing.

All the good recovery stories I have just cited were all with synthetic vitamin C. It simply isn't possible to find the therapeutic high doses I have described from natural sources. So there is no question that synthetic vitamin C does the same job, or better.

What I did find, though, was that the manufactured source of vitamin C could cause unpleasant allergic reactions. The most common starting point is corn, so a sensitive corn-allergic individual could react to it.

But other plant sources are available, such as palm. These would be safer.

Throughout this section, I'll be referring to the D3 form (cholecalciferol or calciol), which has powerful immune booster properties. Without doubt D is the most powerful immune booster vitamin we know. It is highly effective at reducing mortality from all causes (recent 2007 studies). It lowers the cancer risk by over 60%. You want to be taking adequate amounts as of now. Don't wait for an emergency.

In April 2005, a virulent strain of influenza hit a maximum-security forensic psychiatric hospital for men that's midway between San Francisco and Los Angeles. John J. Cannell, a psychiatrist there, observed with increasing curiosity as one infected ward after another was quarantined to limit the outbreak. Although 10 percent of the facility's 1,200 patients ultimately developed the flu's fever and debilitating muscle aches, none did in the ward that he supervised. Even though they had mingled with patients from infected wards before their quarantine, none developed the illness.

A few months later, Cannell ran across a possible answer in the scientific literature. In the July 2005 FASEB Journal (Federation of American Societies for Experimental Biology), an article reported that vitamin D boosts production in white blood cells of one of the antimicrobial compounds that defends the body against germs.

Immediately, Cannell realized, the high doses of vitamin D that he had been prescribing to virtually all the men on his ward were the reason for the mass immunity.

Vitamin D stimulates cathelicidin production. The cathelicidins are an important group of antimicrobial proteins. They work by punching holes in the external membrane of a microbe, permitting its innards to leak out. They also trigger the congregation of white cells when we get an infection.

You can think of these as "on-board" antibiotics; part of our innate immunity.

The FASEB Journal article also triggered Cannell's recollection that children with rickets, a hallmark of vitamin D deficiency, tend to experience more infections than do kids without the bone disease. He shared his flu data with some well-known vitamin D researchers, and they urged him to investigate further.

On the basis of more than 100 articles that he collected, Cannell and seven other researchers now propose that vitamin D deficiency may underlie a vulnerability to infections by the microbes that cathelicidin targets. These include bacteria, viruses, and fungi, the group notes in a report available online for the December 2006 Epidemiology and Infection.

This is only a hypothesis, "but a very credible one" My take on this too is that the population malnutrition I was referring to in the previous sections, which was the main reason the infectious diseases declined, could be as much due to improved vitamin D status as other factors.

Scientists are beginning to suspect that would hold true for the decline in TB, also. A study published in 2006 investigated the relationship between vitamin D and susceptibility to tuberculosis and showed dramatically better recovery in patients supplemented with 10,000 IU daily. 100% of patients survived, while normally 40 - 50% will die, despite treatment *[Acta Med Indones. 2006 Jan-Mar;38(1):3-5]*

Maybe vitamin D status is the MAIN reason we fight infections better when we are properly nourished. In any case, the moral is clear: don't let yourself be deficient.

This article in the prestigious New England Journal Of Medicine made it clear that cathelicidn defiency was associated with increased susceptibility to Staph. infections (hence MRSA) *[Ong, P. Y., Ohtake, T., Brandt, C., Strickland, I., Boguniewicz, M., Ganz, T., Gallo, R. L. & Leung, D. Y. (2002) N. Engl. J. Med. 347, 1151-1160.]*

Ignore stupid and criminal government advice here in the USA and take at least 1,000 units a day. 2,000- 5,000 units would make more sense in an epidemic or if you are battling MRSA.

Vitamin D Cream

Vitamin D as a cream may have important potential for those with MRSA of the skin.

Independently, dermatologist Mona Ståhle of the Karolinska Institute in Stockholm reached a similar conclusion. Her team administered an ointment containing a drug mimic of 1,25-D to the skin of four healthy people. The salve hit "the jackpot, right away," Ståhle says. In the May 2005 Journal of Investigative Dermatology, her team reported that where the ointment had been applied, cathelicidin-gene activity skyrocketed as much as 100-fold.

The team also found evidence of a localized increase in the concentration of cathelicidin.

Scientists found that vitamin D was also effective against TB. The sunlight/vitamin D effect might explain why blacks are racially more prone to TB. It would also tell us one reason why the sanitoriums, with their keen emphasis on fresh air and sunshine, had some measurable therapeutic results, even before the days of hospitalization.

120 or so reports over the past 70 years have pointed to a link between vitamin D and resistance to infections. Five studies since the 1930s that have linked reduced risks of infectious disease to dietary supplementation with cod liver oil, a rich source of vitamin D.

Just think about what you do know for a moment--- in winter, colds, flu, and other respiratory diseases are more common and more likely to be deadly than they are in summer. During winter, ultraviolet-light exposure tends to be low because people spend more time indoors and the atmosphere filters out more of the sun's rays, especially at mid and high latitudes.

Sun exposure—in moderation—might also prove therapeutic, Ståhle's team suggested in the November 2005 Journal of Investigative Dermatology. The scientists showed that in eight fair-skinned people, a single dose of ultraviolet-B radiation—just enough to evoke some skin reddening the next day—activated the vitamin D receptor and the cathelicidin gene in the exposed skin.

This reminds me that in preantibiotic days, tuberculosis patients were put on a fresh-air-and sunshine regimen. Could the vitamin D so acquired account for the cures this system sometimes produced?

Take a minimum of 2,000 IU a day, double or treble that in an epidemic. Ignore official advice that you don't need more than 200 IU a day. It will kill you. A tablespoon has around 1400- 1500 IU.

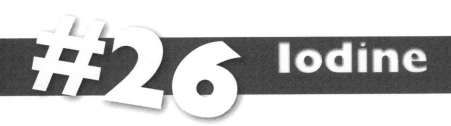

#26 Iodine

Here's a much neglected mineral deficiency that has profound effects on the performance of the immune system.

According to the WHO, 2.2 billion people worldwide are at risk for Iodine Deficiency Disease. Iodine deficiency impairs immune function. The myth that it only affects people in areas remote from the sea is made nonsense by these figures. Deficiency is everywhere. According to Dr David Brownstein iodine intake in the USA has fallen by 50% during the last 30 years.

We had iodized table salt but any intelligent doctor can see the clear evidence that iodine is not absorbed from salt. It was iodine in bread that actually helped the problem. But 30 years ago manufacturers ceased adding iodine to bread and instead used bromine, which counteracts iodine! Any wonder then?

Test For Iodine Deficiency

Dip a cotton bud in iodone solution, such as Lugol's or tincture of iodine and make a patch on your skin. If the yellowish stain disappears in less than an hour; it means your body is lacking crucial iodine and has soaked it up. If the stain remains for more than four hours, you iodine levels are fine.

Iodine levels are not just important for immunity. Low levels of iodine will impair thyroid function. Since the thyroid too is involved in the immune response, it's a double-whammy for your immune system if you are low.

If there is an epidemic pending or occurring, get yourself plenty of iodine fast. When times are safer, be more concerned about regulating the dose

Remember, women are naturally prone to iodine deficiencies. That's because the thyroid gland in women is twice as large as in men -- so under normal circumstances, women need more iodine. However, when there is increased stress (and when is a woman's life not stressful?), the need for iodine can double or triple.

Take 5 mg a day minimum, start now, don't wait for infections to strike. Ignore claims that iodine is toxic. So is anything if you take too much. The necessary doses are 10- 50 times higher than fashions claim. One of the best ways to boost your iodine levels is to add seaweed sea vegetables to your diet. Just one teaspoon of sea vegetables a day can help you regain normal iodine levels. Incorporating seafood and fish into your diet can also help. Other foods that contain iodine are eggs and dairy products, including milk, cheese and yogurt, onions, radishes, and watercress. Some foods, called goitrogens, should be omitted for a while as they hinder iodine utilization.

These included kale, cabbage, peanuts, soy flour, Brussels sprouts, cauliflower, broccoli, kohlrabi and turnips.

Tincture of iodine is often found in emergency survival kits, used both to disinfect wounds and to sanitize surface water for drinking.

When an alcohol solution is not desirable, Lugol's iodine, an aqueous solution of iodine in potassium iodide solution, or povidone iodine (Betadine), a PVPI solution, can be used.

When using free iodine to sanitize surface water, it should be left to sit for 30 minutes before drinking, allowing time for all viruses and bacteria to be killed. If the water temperature is less than 20 °C (68 °F), sitting time should be extended to several hours. To purify 1 L (34 oz) of water, 0.3 mL (0.01 oz) of 2% tincture should be used. Cold or cloudy water should be given 2.4 mL (0.08 oz) of 2% iodine, and should be left to sit for several hours.

Following disinfection, the iodine odor and taste can be removed by adding powdered vitamin C, which converts the iodine to iodide. A similar reaction also removes chlorine from chlorinated water.

Iodine used to sanitize water is also available in tablet or crystal form. One form or another should be available at health stores, and trip outfitters.

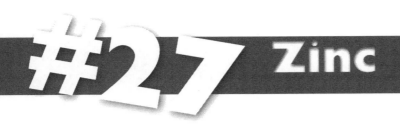

Who doesn't know that zinc helps fight infection? It also helps with wound repair and a number of other key healing functions.

Zinc is an essential mineral that is naturally present in some foods, added to others, and available as a dietary supplement. Zinc is also found in many cold lozenges and some overthe-counter drugs sold as cold remedies.

Zinc is involved in numerous aspects of cellular metabolism. It is required for the proper functioning of approximately 100 enzymes and it plays a role in immune function, protein synthesis, wound healing, DNA synthesis and cell division.

The critical point to note is that a daily intake of zinc is required to maintain a steady state because the body has no specialized zinc storage system. Yet our diets are notoriously lacking in zinc. Studies show that an average diet does not meet the recommended requirements (15 mg daily).

Partly it is removed in the processing of food, especially in refining grains. Phytate inhibition further reduces the bio-availability of zinc. To make matters worse, crops grown in Europe and the US may be short of zinc because the soil has become exhausted.

Signs of a lack of zinc are said to be white flecks in the finger nails and an impaired sense of taste. Professor Bryce-Smith's zinc status test rests on the fact that zinc-deficient individuals cannot taste the metal in solution as zinc sulphate. After adequate supplementation, taste appears to return.

Zinc works in concert with other vitamins and co-enzymes. For example, vitamin A metabolism needs zinc. B6, so helpful in many conditions, is far more effective in the presence of zinc and magnesium. Zinc appears to counteract copper and an imbalance of the ratio of these two metals is associated with an increased tendency to allergies.

Zinc supplements reduce the average duration of the common cold. Other clues suggest the importance of zinc in immunity.

Supplements

Zinc is available in a large number of proprietary preparations such as in the gluconate or orotate form. Doses of around 15 mg are required, but beware: quoted weights usually include the whole formula. A tablet with 100 mg of zinc as gluconate may have only 2 mg of elemental zinc!

Research has not determined whether differences exist among forms of zinc in absorption, bioavailability, or tolerability. However I recall a paper suggesting that the citrate form is best absorbed. For cheapness and convenience I often give zinc sulfate as a powder, 7 g dissolved in a pint of water. The patient takes a teaspoon per day of this liquid, providing about 15 mg daily.

In addition to standard tablets and capsules, some zinc-containing cold lozenges are labeled as dietary supplements.

Ironically, after what I said about the returning sense of smell, there have been several case reports of anosmia (permanent loss of smell) from the use of zinc-containing nasal gels or sprays, and so this raises questions about the safety of intranasal zinc.

Health Risks from Excessive Zinc

Zinc toxicity can occur in both acute and chronic forms. Acute adverse effects of high zinc intake include nausea, vomiting, loss of appetite, abdominal cramps, diarrhea, and headaches. Intakes of 150 - 450 mg of zinc per day have been associated with such chronic effects as low copper status, altered iron function, reduced immune function, and reduced levels of high-density lipoproteins. Reductions in a copper-containing enzyme, a marker of copper status, have been reported with even moderately high zinc intakes of approximately 60 mg/day for up to 10 weeks.

Therefore I do not recommend that you exceed 15- 20 mg a day of elemental zinc.

However- it may not be that simple.

Although zinc is clearly needed for competent T-cell mediated immunity, it has the opposite effect on neutrophils and macrophages, causing a reduction in their motility and ability to ingest invaders. That could explain a recent cautionary finding: that zinc may favor the growth and activity of bacteria over the cells of the host (rather like excess iron, see next section).

In an article appearing in the Dec. 1 2008 online edition of Proceedings of the National Academy of Sciences, researchers in UC's department of molecular genetics, biochemistry and microbiology detailed findings that the presence of zinc is crucial to the formation of infection-causing biofilms.

Staphylococci can grow as biofilms, which are specialized communities of bacteria that are highly resistant to antibiotics and immune responses. They are remarkably adhesive and can grow on many surfaces, including implanted medical devices such as pacemakers, heart valve replacements and artificial joints. Preventing or inhibiting the growth of such biofilms would dramatically reduce the incidence of staph infections.

UC researchers in the lab of Andrew Herr, PhD, found that zinc causes a protein on the bacterial surface to act like molecular Velcro, allowing the bacterial cells in the biofilm to stick to one another. Zinc chelation, or removal, prevented biofilm formation by Staphylococcus epidermidis and Staphylococcus aureus.

So zinc is a definite immune booster but has the surprising effect of favoring staphylococci and other invaders. Stay tuned for updates.

Here's where nutrition gets tricky, even dangerous. Excess iron in the human body causes fulminating fatalities, whenever there are serious bacterial infections. Iron favours the invader far more than the immune system.

The public has it so hammered into them that virtually everyone is iron deficient and "Better take some extra, just to be safe". This is the grossest nutritional mistake that is made by ignorant or foolish MDs today. Iron EXCESS is far from rare and is very dangerous indeed. If you have it and land in an epidemic or pandemic, you are for it!

Did you know that patients with iron overload disease are told not to walk on beaches barefoot? This is on account of a bacterium common in all sea water called Vibrio vulnificus. This bacterium, when it encounters stored iron in our bodies, becomes catastrophically toxic in the presence of excess iron. But how common is iron overload disease?

About 20% of the population is in danger. There are 42 million people at risk from iron overload in the U. S. population alone. Some population segments such as the Scott/Irish and the African Americans have twice the double gene frequency and an amazing 20% carrier rate in the U.S.

You may be risking your health if you take otc multi vitamins or minerals with iron or vitamin C without knowing your iron storage status. Vitamin C has been found to mobilize stored iron into the heart muscle where it sets up arrhythmia or heart rhythm disturbances. It can also cause people to over absorb iron even from their ordinary diets. Do not take vitamin C supplements if you have, or might have this condition, until you have found out for sure.

Meanwhile stupid or ignorant doctors go on prescribing iron pills (huge doses around 250 mgm) as if they were sweeties and not a compound which is more lethal than arsenic to millions of people!

Never mind iron deficiency; it is much more important to know if someone is in iron overload.

Maybe you are? Two lab tests will settle it: Transferrin saturation. Serum Iron (SI) divided by Total Iron Binding Capacity (TIBC) and Serum Iron (SI) gives Transferrin Saturation TS. It should be 12-45%.

Serum Ferritin. Normal range is: 5 to 150.

Without being in possession of this important laboratory information, remember you have a 1:5 risk of iron overload and you will die very swiftly if a plague of any organism does occur. Get it fixed before the problem occurs (the cure is chelation or, in an emergency, blood letting).

Overleaf there's a picture of what vibrio vulnificus did to one man's leg, just before the amputation. I DON'T RECOMMEND YOU LOOK AT THIS, UNLESS YOU HAVE A GOOD STOMACH.

This is a man who went fishing one day, got a tiny scratch on his leg and just wiped the blood off. This bacteria moves fast. He complained next morning about tightness in the leg and was running a fever that evening and he all but died that night in agonizing pain that no meds could relieve.

The irony is he never even got out of the boat.

I urge you to take all care, get your iron levels checked now and learn EVERYTHING you can about antibiotic substitutes. Get rid of any MD who scoffs. Find a good one.

Doctor's do not give warnings about vulvificus to immune compromised patients (Kidney, Liver, Hepatitis C, Cancer, Leukemia, immune suppressant drugs, the list is long). If that applies to you, stay out of the water on the Gulf Coast between April and October.

Remember: vulnificus can enter the body through a tiny cut or bite. If you must go fishing, take with you a bucket filled with bleach water or hydrogen peroxide and dip your hands in it several times an hour.

If you suspect you (or a loved one) got unlucky, use the MMS protocol immediately, while en route to the hospital.

We hear about tropical rainforests and the medicinal wonders they produce. Actually the ordinary garden also contains many such substances, as some of you may know.

Even conventional medicine is getting on to this; 20 years ago kids with leukemia were in trouble; 4 out of 5 died. Now it's 4 out of 5 survive, thanks to the periwinkle plant (Vinca major). This humble little ground cover plant has given us vinblastine and vincristine, two very powerful chemo agents.

But really, when we say "herbs", we usually mean gentler phytotherapies than this!

Probably the most famous herb for beating infections is Echinacea (Coneflower). It's not the best, in my opinion, but certainly deserves a favorable mention. It fortifies the immune system.

But I find the results of using just this herb disappointing. Moreover numerous clinical trials have failed to show much positive effect. Not all studies are corrupt and bent only on rubbishing natural therapies! I would not ask anyone to rely much on Echincea as protection in an epidemic or real pandemic.

The best way to take Echinacea is as a homeopathic compound. I have in mind one product in particular, which is Echinacea compositum, by the German manufacturer HEEL. It's best taken as liquid vials: if no doctor is available to administer it IV, a patient can still take the ampoules, one dissolved in water every third day (one day ON, two days OFF).

There are other immune fortifying herbs, such as Astragalus, Boneset, Calendula, Lady's Mantle (Alchemilla) and Yarrow. Ginger has powerful anti-infective, anti-parasitic, and anti-inflammatory properties.

Compare these also with the benefits of fungi and mushrooms, described in another section (#38).

Thing is, herbs have a place but I wouldn't really rely on them if an infection was raging in my body. I'd want something that killed bacteria (bactericidal) or at least held them down while the immune system got to work beating them to death (bacteriostatic)!

There are some plant sources which are definitely powerful antibiotics. They hold in check, and even kill, bacteria.

Best-known by far, of course, is common garlic. Some others are probably better.

We can use herbs in a variety of ways, apart from just eat them. For example, herbal infusions, herbal baths and herbal wraps, as well as dried leaf powders and capsules.

Then there is essential oil therapy. This, as you will see in a later section, is very different from recreational "aromatherapy". Essential oils were in fact the first serious antibiotics that we had in the 20th century. These oils are still there and still work. Doctors ignore them but that doesn't mean they are not to be preferred to synthetic manufactured compounds with complicated side effects!

Herbs can also be smoked! I found this study on PubMed from the Department of Pharmacy and Pharmacology, Faculty of Health Sciences, University of the Witwatersrand in South Africa (Abstract): "Validation Of Smoke Inhalation Therapy To Treat Microbial Infections."

Aim Of The Study: In traditional healing, the burning of selected indigenous medicinal plants and the inhalation of the liberated smoke are widely accepted and a practiced route of administration. This study elucidated the rationale behind this commonly practiced treatment by examining the antimicrobial activity of five indigenous South African medicinal plants commonly administered through inhalation (Artemisia afra, Heteropyxis natalensis, Myrothamnus flabellifolius, Pellaea calomelanos and Tarchonanthus camphoratus).

Material And Methods: An apparatus was designed to simulate the burning process that occurs in a traditional setting and the smoke fraction was captured for analysis and bioassay. Methanol and acetone extracts as well as the essential oil (for the aromatic species) were prepared and assayed in parallel with the smoke fraction.

Results: Antimicrobial data revealed that in most cases, the 'smoke-extract' obtained after burning had a better effect than the corresponding solvent extracts and essential oils. So the "smidging" tradition of the North American indians was validated.

The report concluded that "These results suggest that the combustion process produces an 'extract' with superior antimicrobial activity and provides in vitro evidence for inhalation of medicinal smoke as an efficient mode of administration in traditional healing."

[J Ethnopharmacol. 2008 Oct 28;119(3):501-6. Epub 2008 Aug 19.]

Homeopathy: Section #41

Finally, don't forget that many homeopathic remedies (section 41) are also derived from herbs and have similar or related properties.

#30 Calendula

This plant sits halfway between the immune fortifiers and actual antibiotic herbs. It has a definite antispectic action and a measurable antibiotic action. It's great for minor skin infections, such as wounds and abcesses.

Calendula officinalis (pot marigold) comes from Latin and means "the first day of the month". This wonderful annual, which grows up to 28 inches tall, produces cheerful flowers that have a faint but distinctive scent. Its leaves can be added to salads while the flowers add a colorful garnish to many dishes (some people even eat the garnish!)

Medicinal Calendula preparations are usually made from either the whole flower heads or just the petals. The flower head contains an essential oil that has an antibiotic effect and lends the flower its characteristic scent. Other components include calendon, which also has a strong odor, and a carotene-like dye calendulin.

Calendula works well as a fairly strong antiseptic properties both topically and internally. Applied externally to the skin, the plant's antibiotic action helps promote the painless healing of minor wounds by reducing inflammation and pus formation.

I've prescribed calendula ointment for decades as a burn remedy. It helps keep the wound antiseptic and promotes healing without scarring.

Calendula can also be used as a gargle to relieve sore throats.

Making Calendula tea:

Pour 1 cup of boiling water over 1-2 tsp. of dried calendula petals. Steep for 10 min, then strain. Drink 2-3 cups of warm tea daily. Use as a gargle for sore throats.

For immediate dressing of wounds pluck (or buy) fresh flowers and squeeze to extract the juice, which you can apply directly to wounds.

Calendula ointment can be bought in stores or prepared at home by mixing a few drops of calendula oil with skin lotion. Apply it to minor burns, bruises, cuts and scrapes. The homeopathic form of Calendula is best taken as 30C tablets. So-called homeopathic Calendula ointment is also available but at 1X (ten times diluted) it's hardly homeopathic. It cost just a few dollars.

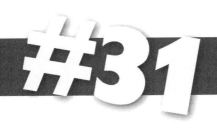

#31 Garlic

It was used by the ancient Egyptians, Chinese, the Greeks and Romans. In 1858, Louis Pasteur demonstrated the powerful antibacterial properties of garlic. It was used in both World Wars. When no other antiseptic or antibiotic was available wounds were smeared with crushed garlic juice and then bandaged. In WW2 the Russians used it when antibiotic supplies ran out. It was called "Russian Penicillin".

Modern research has shown that garlic juice can slow the growth of (and even kill) more than 60 species of mould, and more than 20 species of bacteria, including some that are very virulent. It is also currently attracting attention because of its ability to lower blood pressure, cholesterol, and for its possible anti-cancer properties.

The active ingredients are ajoene and allicin. Ajoene breaks down via sulfenic acid to allicin when it is crushed. Allicin is the chief antibiotic compound. Allicin gives rise to the characteristic garlic smell. Don't be fooled by sales talk that garlic oil and capsules have the same effect as raw, stinky garlic!

1 mgm of allicin is said to be equivalent to 15 standard units of penicillin. The standard dose of penicillin is around 1500 Units, so 100 mgms of allicin could be equivalent to a penicillin dose!

There are over 2,000 studies on the antibiotic efficacy of garlic.

Microbiologist Dr Ron Cutler, based at the University of East London, claims that the garlic compound allicin not only kills established varieties of MRSA, but also destroys the new generation of 'super-superbugs' that have evolved resistance to Vancomycin and Glycopeptides, the powerful antibiotics widely considered to be the last line of defence against MRSA.

Allicin can cure patients with MRSA-infected wounds within weeks, according to in vitro research presented at the Institute of Biomedical Scientists congress in Birmingham during October 2003 and was published in the Journal of Biomedical Science 2004.

[Cutler, RR; P Wilson (2004). "Antibacterial activity of a new, stable, aqueous extract of allicin against methicillan-resistant Staphylococcus aureus (PDF file)". British Journal of Biomedical Science 61 (2): 71-4. http://www. allimax.us/Cutler.pdf. Retrieved on 20 Feb 2009.]

After showing that allicin destroys the MRSA microbe in laboratory trials, Cutler has now teamed up with the firm Allicin International to develop topical treatments including a nasal cream, oral capsules and soaps that have proved effective against both MRSA and GISA.

Another study published in 2002 found that raw garlic consumption could help limit the dam-age done to the heart after surgery because of its natural antioxidant properties. Supplements of allicin have also been shown to reduce risk of colds, prevent high blood pressure and kill cancer cells. So eat it!

Garlic may be one of the reasons the so-called Mediterranean diet prolongs life; it includes lots of garlic, fresh and cooked. If you are not used to using this amazing plant flavor, it's time you got it into your diet.

Just make sure some of it is raw, chopped up or blended in sauces and salsas etc. Cooked garlic has little of the properties it is famous for.

Kyolic is aged garlic and rather different but a powerful medicinal in its own right.

Note: garlic can interfere with the action of some anticoagulant drugs.

Use Garlic Tea as an Antibiotic

Here's how to make it: Place a few cloves of garlic, pre-crushed, into a saucepan of water and bring it to a boil.

Remove the pan from the heat. Stir in the honey and lemon juice or a little of some other suitable sweetener, such as maple syrup.

Strain into a warmed teapot and sip about half a cup.

Repeat 3 times a day, either hot or cold. Refrigerate the remaining tea.

Surface Application: In an emergency it can be crushed and the juice applied to the site of an open wound to kill bacteria such as staph and strep. These strains of bacteria cannot become immune to garlic's effect as it has modern synthesized antibiotics because garlic kills in a different way.

Better Than Garlic? I Think So!

Artemisia is a large, diverse genus of plants with between 200 to 400 species belonging to the daisy family Asteraceae. It comprises hardy herbs and shrubs known for their volatile oils. They grow in temperate climates of the Northern Hemisphere and Southern Hemisphere, usually in dry or semi-dry habitats. The fern-like leaves of many species are covered with white hairs.

It is said that the genus Artemisia (which includes over 400 plants) may be named after an ancient botanist. Artemisia was the wife and sister of the Greek/Persian King Mauseolus (from whose name we get the word mausoleum). Artemisia, who ruled for three years after the king's death, was a botanist and medical researcher, and died in 350 B.C. *(Wikipedia)*.

The two best known plants are Artemisia annua (Sweet Wormwood, Sweet Annie, Sweet Sagewort or Annual Wormwood. Chinese : pinyin) and Artemisia absinthum. The latter has no significant medicinal properties and is the basis of the drink absinthe. It has been banned in many countries, for its brain-rotting effects.

Vermouth (from the German Wermut) was originally made with wormwood but now uses more innocent herbs for flavor.

Other members of this family include the cooking herb Tarragon.

Most members of the genus are bitter. This led to the plant being used by wet-nurses for weaning infants from the breast, as in this speech by Shakespeare from Romeo and Juliet Act I, Scene 3:

Nurse: ...   And she [Juliet] was wean'd, – I never shall forget it, –   Of all the days of the year, upon that day: For I had then laid wormwood to my dug, ...

Scientific Interest

There is a lot of interest in the medical properties of Artemisia annua, which I shall call simply Artemisia from this point. Its chief ingredient, artemisinin, is a potent anti-malarial, anti-fungal and even anti-cancer substance. A search of PubMed with the term artemsinin yields hundreds of papers.

Artemisinin is a terpene which contains peroxide bridges. Taken along with section #19 on hydrogen peroxide this can be seen why it would benefit infections, even including the very difficult case of toxoplasma cysts.

Two other important active ingredients which are widely being studied are artesunate and artemether. They seem to have pretty good anti-infective properties too. To quote a study carried out at the Centre for Infection, Division of Cellular and Molecular Medicine, University of London, and published in the journal Trends in Pharmacological Science [Trends Pharmacol Sci. 2008 Oct;29(10):520-7]:

"Artemisinins are derived from extracts of sweet wormwood (Artemisia annua) and are well established for the treatment of malaria, including highly drug-resistant strains. Their efficacy also extends to phylogenetically unrelated parasitic infections such as schistosomiasis. More recently, they have also shown potent and broad anticancer properties in cell lines and animal models. In this review, we discuss recent advances in defining the role of artemisinins in medicine, with particular focus on their controversial mechanisms of action. This safe and cheap drug class that saves lives at risk from malaria can also have important potential in oncology."

Malaria

Artemisinin has become well-known for its powerful anti-malarial effect. At a time when the world is steadily losing control of the disease, due to widespread drug resistance of the malaria parasite Plasmodium falciparum.

Systematic reviews on Artemisinin show that it is as effective as quinine in treating both uncomplicated and severe malaria. Unfortunately, the relapse rate was still high when used alone.

But artemisinin in conjunction with a suitable anti-biotic, a protocol called "Artemisia combination therapy" (ACT), has been found to be highly effective. Coartem, from artemisinin combined with an antibiotic lumefantrine, wipes out malaria in more than 96 percent of patients in regions where malaria has become resistant to older drugs. Traditional meds such as chloroquine work in only 50 percent of patients where the parasite is drug-resistant. There were an estimated 247 million malaria cases in 2006, and nearly 881,000 patients died, according to the World Health Organization.

Coartem was approved by the Swiss in the late 1990s and put on the World Health Organization (WHO) essential drug list in 2002. The USA was typically way behind world progress, with the FDA holding it back till early 2009 (the USA mistakenly believes only their doctors and scientists are competent to make these decisions).

Other Pathogens

To be included in this report Artemisia would have to affect more than just malaria, though this disease is actually the world's number one killer.

I found a paper which showed artemisinin in combination with ampicillin or unasyn (a complex of ampicillin and sulbactam) decreased mortality in mice subjected to a lethal live E. coli challenge from 100 to 66.7% or 33.3%, respectively [Antimicrob Agents Chemother. 2006 July; 50(7): 2420–2427].

It seems clear it has widespread anti-biotic applications. Studies published on the Sloan-Kettering website show anti-parasitic properties. In vitro studies indicate that artemisinin may be an effective treatment for other protozoal infections such as leishmaniasis, Chagas' disease, and African sleeping sickness. [http://www.mskcc.org/mskcc/html/69126.cfm, accessed June 27th 2009, 10.40 am PST]

Another study from the University of Nizwa, Oman, showed in vitro antimycoplasmal activity of six Jordanian medicinal plants, including a related Artemisia, against three Mycoplasma species. Trop Anim Health Prod. 2007 Oct;39(7):515-9.Links All Mycoplasma species showed susceptibility to Artemisia herba-alba and Artemisia arborescens with MIC ranges from 3.125-12.5 mg/ml.

Incidentally, this study compared garlic and pomegranate with Artemisia arborescens and showed they had only limited activity against some Mycoplasma isolates.

Another Artemisia was helpful with Helicobacter pylori, the scourge of stomach ulcers (and stomach cancer). Increasing drug resistance means we are now losing ground in this "breakthrough" treatment of ulcers. Artemisia may be the answer.

A study in Mexico published in the Journal of Ethnopharmacology showed Artemisia ludoviciana (also Persea americana, Annona cherimola, Guaiacum coulteri, and Moussonia deppeana) had high antHelicobacter pylori. *[J Ethnopharmacol. 2009 Mar 18;122(2):402-5].*

How To Take It

The good news is that it is free. Artemisia annua flourishes in almost any garden, worldwide.

A 2004 test reported that Artemisinin is absorbed faster from the tea preparations than from capsules. The maximum plasma concentrations were observed after 30 minutes. Artesunate is rapidly absorbed and reaches maximum plasma level within 45-90 minutes *[Rath K, et al. Pharmacokinetic study of artemisinin after oral intake of a traditional preparation of Artemisia annua L. (annual wormwood). Am J Trop.Med Hyg. 2004;70:128-32].*

Making The Tea: One litre (2 pints) of boiling water is poured onto 5 g dried leaves (large tablespoonful, loose, or teaspoon if crushed to a powder) of Artemisia annua. It is allowed to brew for 10 to 15 minutes, and then poured through a sieve. This tea is then drunk in four portions in the course of the day. The period of treatment is between 5 and 7 days.

Patients with gastrointestinal disorders or those taking antacids should not take Artemisia because it increases the production of stomach acid *[Skyles AJ, Sweet BV. Alternative therapies. Wormwood. Am J Health Syst.Pharm. 2004;61:239-42].*

It is also unwise to use this remedy if you are taking antiseizure medications; Artemisia can induce seizures resulting in decreased efficacy of antiseizure medications [previous reference].

You may not have heard of this powerful antibacterial and anti-inflammatory. It's in the Cats Claw family but reputedly 1,000 times stronger in its immune enhancing effect than ordinary Cats Claw.

Samento is the name given to the plant by the Ashaninka Indians in the Peruvian rainforest. They have ancient knowledge of the plant and use it for a wide variety of complaints.

The Indians are a crucial source of the plant materials because they can recognize the correct strain, without the need do elaborate tests. Let me explain why this is important:

Ordinary Cats Claw contains important oxidole alkaloids, one of the many important groups of phyto-nutrients found in the plant. One strain of plants contains pentacyclic oxindole alkaloids (POAs); the other contains both POAs and tetracyclic oxindole alkaloids (TOAs).

POAs act on the cellular immune system and TOAs act on the central nervous system. TOAs are not good because they interfere with the benefits of the POAs. This is confirmed by studies.

Uncaria tomentosa plants may contain as much as 80% TOAs. According to studies in Austria, as little as 1% TOAs can cause a 30% reduction in the acquired immune benefits that POAs provide. So even a little TOAs, if present, can go a long way to neutralizing the benefits of Cats Claw.

This explains why lots of the common herb were needed by Western herbalists, to produce any real effect. But the amazing strain found by the Ashaninka Indians does not have the destructive TOAs. Make sure when you buy Samento, that the packet specifically states no TOAs. Otherwise it isn't Samento anyway!

Samento has shown dramatic benefits in virtually every kind of inflammation, such as asthma and arthritis.

It can also fight infections from AIDS to hepatitis' flu to salmonella. Its broad spectrum effect helps to increase T-lymphocyte and microphage production. It also helps repair the lipid matrix in the cell walls and is particularity good for stopping the expansion of virus laden cells.

The 2 active ingredients are berberine and hydrastine. These are good for killing many of the bacteria that cause diarrhea, such as E. Coli, Salmonella, Shigella, Klebsiella and the cholera bacterium. Also parasites like ameba, giardia and trachoma. It also has antifungal properties, so would suit Candida patients. It's even effective to some degree against TB.

Samento may even have anti-cancer action. Renato Rizzi, at the University of Milan, led an experiment with Samento as it relates to cancer causing (mutagenic) substances in smokers. It is well known that the urine of smokers contains mutagenic substances. When given Samento for two weeks, the smoker's urine returned to normal. This is important because it shows Samento may help lessen the risk of developing cancers and other degenerative diseases.

Dose: all these benefits can be had on a dose of just 3 to 6 capsules a day (good for people who hate swallowing lots of tablets and capsules).

#34 Tea Tree
(Melaleuca alternifolia)

I put this plant substance here, though it could just as easily slot into the aromatherapy section coming up.

The plant was named tea tree after Captain James Cook set foot on the shores of Australia back in 1770. The story goes that Cook brewed up a tea from the leaves of the Melaleuca tree and liked it. It has been used for centuries as an antiseptic by the aborigines.

In 1933, the world-class British Medical Journal described Tea Tree Oil as a powerful disinfectant, non-poisonous and non-irritant. In 1930 the Australian Medical Journal reported extremely good results when using tea tree oil to treat everything from septic wounds to scar regeneration. The report stated that the oil dissolved pus, leaving wounds clean without any apparent damage to the tissues.

In 1937 the same journal noted that blood, pus or other organic matter actually increased the antiseptic properties of tea tree oil by about 10-12%. The Australian Government issued little bottles of Tree Oil in the first aid kits of soldiers serving in the tropical regions during the Second World War. In 1955 by the way the United States dispensaries still had Tea tree oil listed as an active germicidal, with an antiseptic action 11 to 30 times more strong than carbolic acid (phenol).

Tea tree oil is very complex, containing over 100 complex chemical components called terpenes (these are what give it its powerful pine-odor). These terpenes make up 80 to 90 percent of the oil.

Tea tree oil is known to be active against many bacteria, including streptococci, staph, E. coli, and various fungi, such as Candida. In a study of 30 patients who had infections that were resistant to a common antibiotic, one-third were completely cured by tea tree oil compared to just 13 percent who received conventional treatment.

Although tea tree oil is seen by the scientific establishment as very much a quaint folk remedy, science is forcing a reexamination of these outdated attitudes towards folk remedies and alternative medicine. Treatments that were once dismissed as nonsense or even quackery, are now been justified through rigorous scientific testing (in facts drugs are often the real quackery and nonsense).

Now I'm going to shock you all and incense thousands of rabid dogmatists in favor of Tea Tree oil, and point out that it may not be what you want at all.

Beware: Tea tree oil may lead to antibiotic resistance

Repeated exposure to low doses of Tea Tree Oil - a common ingredient in many beauty products - can increase the chances of suffering from "superbug" infections, University of Ulster scientists have revealed.

They discovered that exposure to low doses of Tea Tree Oil make pathogens such as MRSA, E. coli and Salmonella more resistant to antibiotics, and capable of causing more serious infections.

Dr Ann McMahon and Professor David McDowell, members of the University's Food Microbiology Research Group, said: "We have been growing pathogens such as MRSA, E-coli and Salmonella in low concentrations of tea tree oil. These concentrations are not sufficient to kill the bacteria, but can switch on their defense mechanisms. Unfortunately, these defense mechanisms have the added effect of making bacteria more resistant to antibiotics, and able to cause "harder to treat" infections."

Tea Tree Oil is used commercially in many products including shampoos, body lotions and toiletries, but there is no legislation requiring manufacturers to state the concentration of tea tree oil in these products.

This increases the risks that people will use low concentrations of tea tree oil, which fail to kill bacteria, but increase their resistance to antibiotics. So, if a person uses tea tree oil products on their skin repeatedly, any MRSA on their skin could develop increased resistance to the antibiotics which are used to control MRSA infections.

"The bottom line is that tea tree oil should not be used at low concentrations - less than 4% - to make sure that bacteria are killed, not just stressed. Otherwise we are just arming the bacteria against treatment by antibiotics."

Publishing their findings in the Journal of Antimicrobial Chemotherapy, the scientists said: "Although tea tree oil may be an effective antimicrobial agent when appropriately used at high (bactericidal) concentrations, its application at low (sub-lethal) concentrations may contribute to the development of antibiotic resistance in human pathogens".

http://www.ulster.ac.uk

The best advice therefore seems to be: if you want to use it, use plenty and make sure you wipe out the bacteria population all at once. Otherwise it's counter productive.

There is one other word of caution too: several cases of gynaecomastia, male breasts in young boys, came about through topical applications of tea tree oil (a shampoo, actually); not many but enough to cause concern.

I pointed this out in one of my publications and was venomously attacked by numerous supposed guardians of "truth". How dare I attack a near sacred old and venerable cure? The mere fact it was hurting young boys was seen as irrelevant. All sorts of arguments were brought forth, including even Robert Tisserand (see Aromatherapy section #39) writing to me and telling me it was probably an estrogenic substance in the plastic shampoo bottles. He didn't even accept that the condition cleared up when the use of the tea tree shampoo was discontinued. It must all be faked propaganda science was his attitude.

Denial is a silly attitude and yet it seems to be almost a requirement to be a card-carrying "holistic therapist". Me? I'd rather stick with at least a semblance of science. All I was asking them was to avoid repeated applications of tea tree in young boys. You'd think I was attacking a sacred cow or even trying to butcher one!

The virtues of Aloe vera have been well known since ancient times. The name was derived from the Arabic alloeh meaning 'bitter' because of the bitter liquid found in the leaves. It is also known as 'lily of the desert', the 'plant of immortality', and the 'medicine plant'.

The fresh gel was said to have been used by Cleopatra to keep her skin soft and young. Aloe vera is truly one of Nature's absolute miracle plants. It seems to be able to cure almost anything. Always think of it with infections, including Candida and yeast.

The outstanding property of Aloe seems to be its gentleness. It is non-irritating and soothes any and all inflammations, whether infective or not. This makes it ideal to take internally and it is also great for vaginal overgrowths, from Candida, to Trich.

If it does seem to be irritating, that is almost certainly due to additives from the manufacturer. If you suspect that, switch to pure Aloe, direct from the plant.

The chief grower and manufacturer of Aloe, worldwide, is an operation called Univera and their flagship product, "Aloe Gold" I highly recommend. I can tell you how to get it, without joining an MLM (admin@informed-wellness.com)

Think of Aloe in situations like dysbiosis, due to excessive use of antibiotics.

It also works as an anthelminthic [an agent that destroys or expels intestinal worms and/or parasites; vermicide; vermifuge]; an antibacterial; an antifungal/yeast; an antiviral and as a parasite treatment.

It may even prevent cancer: that's from the Mayo Clinic website, no less! [http://www.mayo-clinic.com/health/aloe-vera/NS_patient-aloe/DSECTION=evidence]

That's pretty versatile.

Dosage

Adults (18 years and older)

Pure Aloe Vera gel is often used liberally on the skin three to four times per day for the treatment of sunburn and other minor burns. Creams and lotions are also available. There are no reports that using aloe on the skin causes absorption of chemicals into the body that may cause significant side effects. Skin products are available that contain aloe alone or aloe combined with other active ingredients.

For internal use, take 1 – 3 ounces daily.

Children (younger than 18 years)

Topical (skin) use of aloe gel in children is common and appears to be well tolerated. Oral dosing is NOT recommended for kids.

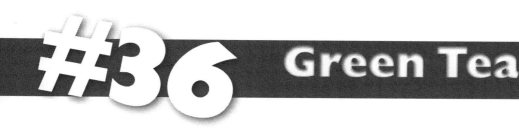

#36 Green Tea

I could, I suppose, have put this with the helpful foods and nutrition section; but I have chosen to feature it in herbs, right after the tea tree!

It may be that green tea can help antibiotics be three times more effective in fighting drug-resistant bacteria, even superbugs. This is according to research at Alexandria University in Egypt, in a paper presented in April 2008 at the Society for General Microbiology in Edinburgh, Scotland.

Green tea is a common drink in Egypt, and that means that many people will drink it while taking antibiotics. The researchers wanted to determine if green tea would help or interfere with the effectiveness of antibiotics. That's reasonable.

"We tested green tea in combination with antibiotics against 28 disease-causing microorganisms belonging to two different classes," Dr Mervat Kaseem, of the university's pharmacy faculty, said in a prepared statement. "In every single case, green tea enhanced the bacteria-killing activity of the antibiotics. For example, the killing effect of chloramphenicol was 99.99 percent better when taken with green tea than when taken on its own in some circumstances."

Kaseem and colleagues also found that green tea made 20 percent of drug-resistant bacteria susceptible to cephalosporin antibiotics, an important type of antibiotics to which new drug-resistant strains of bacteria have evolved resistance.

In almost every case and for all types of antibiotics they tested, the researchers found that drinking green tea at the same time as taking the antibiotics appeared to increase the action of the antibiotics and reduce drug resistance in bacteria. In certain cases, even low concentrations of green tea were effective.

Dr. Kassem has a good point to make: "Our results show that we should consider more seriously the natural products we consume in our everyday life," he said. "In the future, we will be looking at other natural herb products such as majoram and thyme to see whether they also contain active compounds which can help in the battle against drug resistant bacteria."

But wait a minute: I found another study that said we could dispense with the antibiotics altogether! It was carried out for USDA and published in a peer reviewed journal, the Journal of Food Protection. Researchers investigated the antibiotic activity of 11 catechins from green tea and compared these to the strength of 5 medicinal antibiotics.

Their findings and conclusion was startling: three of the catechins beat tetracycline and vancomycin (effective at lower dilutions). I quote: "The results show that three of the catechins exhibited exceptional bactericidal activities at very low levels in the nanomolar range. They were more active than medicinal antibiotics such as tetracycline and vancomycin."

You may remember vancomycin as the "last ditch antibiotic", 30?

So farmers and food suppliers are getting the story, even if your doctor is not!

[Journal of Food Protection. 69:100-107.]

White Tea

But white tea extract seems to be even more powerful, according to a 2004 study conducted at Pace University. Researchers found that White Tea Extract (WTE) may have prophylactic applications in retarding growth of bacteria, viruses and fungi. Their findings were presented at the 104th General Meeting of the American Society for Microbiology.

The anti-viral and anti-bacterial effect of white tea (Stash and Templar brands) is greater than that of green tea. Moreover, the anti-viral and anti-bacterial effect of several toothpastes including Aim, Aquafresh, Colgate, Crest and Orajel was enhanced by the addition of white tea extract.

White tea was more effective than green tea at inactivating bacterial viruses. Results obtained with the bacterial virus, a model system; suggest that WTE may have an anti-viral effect on human pathogenic viruses.

Studies have also indicated that WTE has an anti-fungal effect on Penicillium chrysogenum and Saccharomyces cerevisiae. In the presence of WTE, Penicillium spores and Saccharomyces cerevisiae yeast cells were totally inactivated. It is suggested that WTE may have an anti-fungal effect on pathogenic fungi.

#37 Spices Are Hot Stuff!

Professor Paul W. Sherman and undergraduate student Jennifer Billing prepared a great report on the antibiotic qualities of spices, published in the March 1998 issue of the journal Quarterly Review of Biology.

Sherman credits Billing, a Cornell undergraduate student of biology at the time of the research, with compiling many of the data required to make the microbe-spice connection: More than 4,570 recipes from 93 cookbooks representing traditional, meat-based cuisines of 36 countries; the temperature and precipitation levels of each country; the horticultural ranges of 43 spice plants; and the antibacterial properties of each spice.

Garlic, onion, allspice and oregano were found to be the best all-around bacteria killers (they kill everything), followed by thyme, cinnamon, tarragon and cumin (any of which kill up to 80 percent of bacteria). Capsicums, including chilies and other hot peppers (killed or inhibited up to 75 percent of bacteria), while pepper of the white or black variety inhibits 25 percent of bacteria, as do ginger, anise seed, celery seed and the juices of lemons and limes.

So even mild spices has some measurable effect it seems.

The Cornell researchers noted that in hot countries nearly every meat-based recipe calls for at least one spice, and most include many spices, especially the potent spices, whereas in cooler counties substantial fractions of dishes are prepared without spices, or with just a few." They theorize that spices were a development chiefly intended to inhibit the bacteria of food spoilage.

If that's correct then it is only natural that spices would have a potent antibiotic capacity— and that's what they found.

As decent scientists, they did consider several alternative explanations for spice use and discounted all but one. The problem with the "eat-to-sweat" hypothesis -- that people in steamy places eat spicy food to cool down with perspiration -- is that not all spices make people sweat, Sherman says, "and there are better ways to cool down -- like moving into the shade." The idea that people use spices to disguise the taste of spoiled food, he says, "ignores the health dangers of ingesting spoiled food." However the micronutrient hypothesis -- that spices provide trace amounts of anti-oxidants or other chemicals to aid digestion -- could be true and still not exclude the antimicrobial explanation, Sherman says. However, this hypothesis does not explain why people in hot climates need more micro-nutrients, he adds. The antimicrobial hypothesis does explain this.

"I believe that recipes are a record of the history of the coevolutionary race between us and our parasites. The microbes are competing with us for the same food," Sherman says. "Everything we do with food -- drying, cooking, smoking, salting or adding spices -- is an attempt to keep from being poisoned by our microscopic competitors. They're constantly mutating and evolving to stay ahead of us. One way we reduce food-borne illnesses is to add another spice to the recipe. Of course that makes the food taste different, and the people who learn to like the new taste are healthier for it."

The following are their Top 30 Spices with Antimicrobial Properties (best to least):

1. Garlic

2. Onion

3. Allspice

4. Oregano

5. Thyme

6. Cinnamon

7. Tarragon

8. Cumin

9. Cloves

10. Lemon grass

11. Bay leaf

12. Capsicums

13. Rosemary

14. Marjoram

15. Mustard

16. Caraway

17. Mint

18. Sage

19. Fennel

20. Coriander

21. Dill

22. Nutmeg

23. Basil

24. Parsley

25. Cardamom

26. Pepper (white/black)

27. Ginger

28. Anise seed

29. Celery seed

30. Lemon/lime

Source: "Antimicrobial Functions of Spices: Why Some Like It Hot," Jennifer Billing and Paul W. Sherman, The Quarterly Review of Biology, Vol. 73, No.1, March 1998

Fungi and mushrooms are related to herbal medicines but not quite the same. Remember most antibiotics come from molds, which are related directly to fungi. According to mycologist expert Paul Stamets, fungi are closer to human life than to bacteria. In fact, they too HATE bacteria, which is why they produce powerful antibiotics (bacteria would attack fungi).

The fungi are a remarkable group of organisms that don't need light to synthesize their own food. What we call mushrooms and toadstools are simply the visible fruiting bodies on what is a much larger organism, covering sometimes up to hundreds of square feet, called the mycelium.

The medicinal properties of fungi have been known since ancient times. In fact Oetzi, the "Ice Man" found in the Tyrolean Alps knew about fungi. His body was frozen 5,200 years ago and found to be remarkably preserved when he thawed out after being discovered intact above the 10,000 line in 1991.

His gear was preserved too and that included a medicine pouch, containing a few walnut-sized dried fungi of the species Piptoporus betulinus, known to have antibiotic properties. It shows that Europe was in there with medicinal mushrooms, though not perhaps to the vast extent of Chinese herbal lore.

Now modern science backs up virtually all that has been claimed for mushrooms and fungi. They are immune modulators, anti-viral, antibacterial and anti-cancerous.

Broadly speaking the edible fungi can be divided into those with culinary merits and those which are purely medicinal. There is some overlap; for example, the shiitake mushroom is a well-known Japanese delicacy and has now spread to the West.

Shiitake stimulates the immune system about a hundred times more than the common white button mushroom. Maitake does much more to aid the immune system than morels, portobellos and chanterelles etc. The very tasty oyster mushroom (Pleurotus ostreatus) is an exception and is enjoyed for its antibacterial, anti-viral, blood pressure moderating and cholesterol reducing qualities.

The key to the effectiveness of mushrooms is a substance called beta glucan, a large and complex polysaccharide (sugar chain), which stimulates the immune system to fight pathogens and malignant cells. Maitake is known to be an effective antitumor agent.

Note that yeast beta glucan, commonly sold via MLM networks, is largely ineffective. They love to quote the science but this, if you look closely, is always experiments on the mushroom beta glucan and is NOT applicable to the products they sell (I have a saying: there is science, damned science and then MLM science!)

Mushrooms contain more than just beta glucan, of course: amino acids such as lysine and tryptophan and vitamins such as C, K, nicotinic acid (vitamin B3), riboflavin (B2) pantothenic acid (B5). There are also other complex substances, such as terpenes and steroids.

Reishi

Let's start with the Reishi mushroom (Ganoderma lucidum). To the ancient Chinese this mushroom was called Lingzhi meaning "spirit plant". According to legend, Taoist priests in the first century were supposed to have included the mushroom in magic potions that granted those who consumed them longevity eternal youth and immortality. In Chinese art the Reishi mushroom is a symbol of good health and long life; symbols of it abound everywhere.

Clinical studies have confirmed Reishi has properties as an anti-inflammatory, antioxidant, BP and blood sugar moderator and cholesterol reducer. Reishi contains over 100 bioactive immunomodulatory substances, including beta glucan.

More importantly, studies have shown that Reishi significantly increases three immune signalers known to help the immune system destroy invaders. Japanese researchers say that a hardy system may be able to resist invasions and microbes that weaker host systems may not.

It should also be mentioned that Reishi does not produce some of the negative effects associated with the use of antibiotics, which can often stop the invasion of microbes, but will further weaken the immune response after continued use and are also ineffectual in cases of viruses, pollens and malignant cells.

Maitake

Next let's look at Maitake (Grifola frondosa). Maitake means "dancing mushroom". In Europe it is known as "Hen Of The Woods " and is sometimes called the King Of Mushrooms because of its size.

Maitake is a delicious culinary mushroom but also valued for its medicinal properties. It has known antibiotic activity, although I could only find one really meaningful study to support this. In combination with vancomycin, one of the few remaining antibiotics with some activity against methicillin-resistant Staphylococcus aureus (MRSA), Maitake led to very enhanced survival against Listeria bacteria injected into the abdominal cavity of mice (an often fatal form of food poisoning).

[Kodama N, Yamada M, Nanba H. Jpn J Pharmacol 2001;87:327-332].

Suggested doses: For general protection, 300 mg to 2 grams extract daily, between meals. For therapeutic use against an active infection: 25 to 35 grams extract or more daily until results evident, then taper back to 15 to 30 grams daily, or as recommended by a health care practitioner.

Next, the most famous of all.

Shiitake

It produces a growth inhibiting beta glucan called Lentinan (from shiitake's scientific name Lentinula edodes). Scientists now believe that lentinan and virus-like particles found in shiitake trigger the increased production of various serum factors associated with immunity and inflammation. These so-called lymphokines, such as interferon and interleukin, stimulate the defense system through the proliferation of phagocytes, including macrophages and other immune fighters that attack cancer cells, bacteria, and viruses.

A substance called cortinelin, a broad-spectrum antibacterial agent, which has been isolated from shiitake, kills a wide range of pathogenic bacteria. A sulfide compound extracted from shiitake has been found to have an effect against the fungus that causes ringworm and other skin diseases.

Inonotus obliquus (Chaga)

Stimulates the production of macrophage and NK cells, essential to healthy immune system function. It is rich in immuno-modulating polysaccharides and has been found to be an effective natural anti-inflammatory, anti-tumor, anti-oxidant, anti-viral, and antibiotic.

Pleurotus species

This includes Pleurotus ostreatus (Oyster mushroom). It is enjoyed for its interesting taste, plus anti-bacterial, anti-viral, blood pressure moderating, and cholesterol reducing qualities. It is actually easy to grow at home and is cheap; it should be eaten more widely than it is.

A polycyclic aromatic compound pleurotin has been isolated from P. griseus which possesses antibiotic properties.

Trametes versicolor (Turkey Tail)

Turkey tail mushroom is one of the most widespread mushrooms in the world. Turkey tail can be found on dead trees in just about any hardwood or deciduous forest in North America, Europe, China, Japan and Siberia. As its name indicates, the mushroom looks exactly like a turkey's tail and can be very colorful.

Turkey Tail produces a very powerful immune stimulant polysaccharide, called PSK.

PSK has also been proven as a potent antibiotic, in particular against strains of Staphylococcus aureus, Pseudomonas aeruginosa, Candida albicans, Cryptococcus neoformans, Escherichia coli and Listeria monocytogenes.

[Sakagami, H. & M. Takeda, 1993. "Diverse biological activity of PSK (Krestin): a protein bound polysaccharide from Coriolus versicolor (Fr.) Quel." In Mushroom Biology & Mushroom Products, eds. S.T. Chang J.A. Buswell & Siu-wai Chiu, The Chinese University Press, Hong Kong. pp. 237-245. Mayer, J. & J. Drews, 1980. "The effect of protein-bound polysaccharide from Coriolus versicolor on immunological parameters and experimental infections in mice." Infection 8: 13-21.

Ng, T.B., J.M. Ling, Z.T. Wang, J.N. Cai & G.J. Xu, 1996. "Examination of courmarins, flavonoids and polysaccharopeptides for antibacterial activity." General Pharmacology Oct; 27(7): 1237-40.]

Turkey tail is a little tough to eat so it is usually found in teas, tinctures, capsules and pills.

It just remains to enter a few words of caution:

Firstly, on no account go out and start harvesting mushrooms yourself and trying to make home-brew extracts. You'll likely kill yourself. The Fungi are an enormously large range of organisms and the difference between safe ones and those which kill can be very subtle. It takes an expert to safely identify edible mushrooms. Of course if you live in France or anywhere civilized which really KNOWS food, you can go into any pharmacy and they will identify any mushrooms you gather. But really, you are safer not collecting your own, unless you are a botanist or better still a mycologist (fungologist).

There is an additional problem, which may not be obvious to you, which is getting a predictable dose. It's something which bugs even commercial fungi extracts which you may find for sale on the Net. Let me warn you that the vast majority of products offered are totally worthless, no matter even if the vendor is sincere and well-meaning. It is very difficult to get a regular, effective dose and keep it consistent.

See, part of the difficulty is that fungi are protected by a membrane coat of chitin. That's same stuff insect cases and your fingernails are made of. Just grinding up mushrooms isn't going to get at the best of the content. It needs a heat process to get at the good stuff, by breaking down the chitin. This, of course, is counter-intuitive to most alternative healers and practitioners, who know that heat normally destroys nutrients.

Let me assure you that in this case it's a waste of money, if not extracted properly, and 99% or manufacturers don't even know this, never mind practice it!

To get you over this problem I have identified a range of mushroom products that meet all the necessary requirements for health and effectiveness. They are organically grown, under strict natural conditions, in a special facility Oregon State (which also, incidentally, supplies the WHO with fungal medicines, for treating the populations of Third World Countries). These are the most potent full-spectrum myoceutical products ever produced.

You can get purchase details at:

http://www.powershroom.com

Well, let's move on. Can you see now there is SO MUCH you can do to fight active infections, without the use of antibiotics.

For instance, did you know that essential oils (aromatherapy oils) have powerful antibiotic properties? That was one of their main uses, when first developed. Remember, this was long ago, in the days before antibiotics or any other significant drugs had emerged.

Aromatherapy oils were once not merely for relaxing and getting in touch with the inner self! They were the best pharmaceuticals of the day!

The story goes back a long way, beginning with a man called Chamberla in 1887. He studied a mixture of oregano, cinnamon, angelica and geranium, and he found that each of these inhibited bacteria growth in a petri dish (special culture dish for microbes).

This is exactly the same test that led to the discovery of penicillin. Yet you never hear that these things do essentially the same! Chamberla found the oils very effective against meningococcus (the cause of meningitis), typhus and Staphylococcus (MRSA is a Staphylococcus, remember). But they were not so good against diphtheria and didn't work at all for anthrax—but then, hardly anything ever does.

Another man called Clavell in 1918 showed that clove bud (Syzygium, also a good homeopathic remedy) kills the TB bacillus at 1 part in 6,000. That was an important stepping stone.

In 1928 a famous case was that of Rene-Maurice Gattefosse, who burned his hand. It became infected and smelled very bad. Gattefosse put it in lavender (to ease the smell, presumably) but was surprised when the lavender clearly had a very beneficial effect. He recovered. Gattefosse went on to learn more about plants and their oils and he was the person who invented the term aromatherapy.

In WW2, a French surgeon called Jean Valnet used essential oils to treat injuries and infections and psychiatric disorders. He was able to use these things to treat gangrene successfully. You never get to hear of this today! Nobody ever says that simple herbal oils could be effective against gangrene.

Whoever has been told "You don't need an amputation yet, let's try lavender oil"?

Valnet did a lot of studies and published a book in 1960 called The Practice of Aromatherapy: A Classic Compendium of Plant Medicines and Their Healing Properties.

If you write down Valnet and Aromatherapy and Google that, you will find it. I saw a second-user copy on sale on Amazon for just 5 bucks.

Scientific Testing or Aromatherapy Oils

What astonishes most people (including me, when I first learned it) is that aromatherapy has a good tradition of scientific testing and screening. In the USA it may be looked on askance but in France aromatherapy is quite the thing!

Valnet, in fact, was dedicatedly scientific. He tested numerous plant oils against bacterial culture in petri dishes, exactly the way that led to the discovery of penicillin and other antibiotics. Some were astonishingly good.

1960: Maruzella demonstrated antibacterial and antifungal effects of hundreds of aromatic compounds

1987: Deininger and Lembke demonstrated antiviral activity of essential oils and their isolated components

1973: Wagner and Sprinkmeyer did research on a 170 year old blend of distilled oils still available in Germany. The effects of melissa and the other oils in Kosterfrau Melissengeist had been empirically known since Paracelsus (about 1500). They concluded that, with varying degrees of intensity, there was an inhibiting influence on all the bacteria tested, (Pneumococcus, Klebsiella pneumoniae, Staphlococcus aureus haemolyticus, Neisseria catarrhalis,

Streptococcus haemolyticus, Proteus vulgaris, Hemophilus influenza, Haemophilus pertussis, Candida albicans, Escherichia coli-Aerobacter group, various Corynnebacteria, and Listeria) and stated the large spectrum of this inhibitory action is as broad as or even greater than that of wide-spectrum antibiotics.

One of the most interesting experiments I came across in my research was carried out in the 1960s by Professor Griffon, Director of the French Police Toxicology Laboratory. He researched the use of aromatherapy or essential oils in cleansing the air. Bottom line... dispersing essential oils into the atmosphere dramatically cut down airborne pathogens. After only 30 minutes of airborne spray cultures were down to zero.

He used a mixture of cinnamon, clove, peppermint, lavender, pine, rosemary and thyme.You probably think these are just sissy smells. But actually these are very very powerful substances, I think I will have time to explain these to you before I open for questions.

(This has enormous implications for CA-MRSA ...the respiratory form. If I am not careful, I may run out of time, so let's just do a couple of quick specific...

Drs. Jean-Claude Lapraz and Christian Duraffourd, two Paris-based physicians, organized the world's first phytotherapy conference in Tunisia in May 1993.

Durrafourd and Lapraz have suggested that dosing with essential oils may not be linear in the same way as antibiotics. They found a very small quantity of essential oil had a far greater effect when used in the body than effects measured in vitro (in glass dishes). They also somewhat abandoned the quest for finding one oil for each pathogen. That's something of an allopathic nonsense.

Instead, they see the need for matching the oil to the constitution and make up of the patient in question.

Oregano

Origanum vulgare, also known as Greek or Mediterranean oregano, has good claim to be a natural antibiotic. This is not the cooking oregano however but a rather rare wild herb which grown in the mountainous regions of the eastern Mediterranean. Its scent and flavor are due to the essential oil which has been renowned for its potent antiseptic properties.

When oregano oil was first tested in 1910 it was described as "the most powerful plant-derived antiseptic known" (H. Marindale). It has been found effective both in killing multiple bacteria and preventing their growth. It was shown to be many times more potent than phenol (carbolic acid).

Carvacrol activity crucial. Carvacrol or isopropyl-o-cresol is the active ingredient with powerful antimicrobial properties; it is more potent than carbolic acid.

Oregano has been found to contain several powerful antioxidants such as phenolic acids and flavonoids which protect your tissues against harmful toxins like cancer-causing free radicals *[Tian H, Lai DM. Zhong Yao Cai. 2006;29(9):920-1; Hazzit M, et al. J Agric Food Chem. 2006;54(17):6314-21].*

Oregano oil may be the 'best of the best' among essential oils in killing microbial pathogens, killing bacteria, fungus, yeasts and molds. It was shown to be very effective against Candida (1.5 times more potent than the drug Nystatin).

Specifically, it has activity against:

- Escherichia coli (E. Coli)

- Candida albicans

- Bacillus cereus

- Proteus

- Cryptococcus neoformans

- Staphylococcus aureus (Hence MRSA)

- Streptococcus pneumoniae

- Pseudomonas aerugiosa

- Salmonella

Researchers from the Agricultural Faculty, Selcuk University in Turkey studied essential oils from several different plants, including oregano, laurel, marjoram and mint. They tested these oils on certain bacteria (including Bacillus, which can cause bowel infections and diarrhoea) in the laboratory. All of the herbs, including oregano, were found to successfully block the growth of the bacteria studied *[Ozcan MM, Sagdic O, Ozkan G. J Med Food. 2006 Fall;9(3):418-21].*

In an animal study, performed by scientists at the National Agricultural Research Foundation in Greece, oregano was found to be just as effective as the prescription-only antibiotic neomycin for curing diarrhoea caused by the E.coli bug, which is notorious for causing bowel infections.

Commenting on the findings the scientists said: This study indicates that dried oregano leaves may be as effective in the treatment of coli infection as neomycin *[Bampidis VA, et al. J Vet Med A Physiol Pathol Clin Med. 2006;53(3):154-6]*.

Dose: Oregano oil for products intended for internal use can be used by adding four drops to a small amount of water and take up to three times a day. For external use it can be applied liberally up to three times a day.

Cinnamon

There are two kinds of cinnamon oil, Cinnamomum zeylanicum and Cassia (next section).

Zeylanicum stands for Sri Lanka. I know that because I lived in Sri Lanka for a couple of years. I was professor at a university there. And it's very effective and wonderful to smell. I love it. But it must be said the other cinnamon (Cassia) is more powerful.

A nice idea I found is to make a special flavored honey with this oil:

To 2 oz. of maple syrup or 2 oz. of honey add: 3 drops of Ginger Essential Oil 1 drop Cardamom 1 drop Cinnamon bark oil 3 drops Vanilla Essential Oil, pure 8 drops of certified organic Orange or Mandarin Orange oil

Cassia

Cassia (Cinnamomum cassia, or "hot cinnamon") is native to the south-eastern parts of China and to a lesser extent in Vietnam, Burma and India. It is cheaper and more abundant than the Sri Lanka variety. Its value dependant mainly on the percentage of cinnamic aldehyde which it contains. It is heavier, less liquid, and congeals more quickly than the Ceylonese variety.

Cassia has recognized antimicrobial properties and is often used for diarrhea. The essential oil is a powerful germicide, but being very irritant is rarely used in medicine for this purpose.

One study carried out at the Department of Agricultural Biology and the Research Center for New Bio-Materials in Agriculture, College of Agriculture and Life Sciences, Seoul National University (Koera) showed Cassia had 1/5th - 1/10th the power of tetracycline and chloramphenicol against intestinal bacteria.

Not a problem, since we could always take more Cassia than antibiotic capsules. Interestingly, Cassia had no effect on Lactobacillus, a prime probiotic organism. So there would not be the disastrous after effects of the two antibiotics used in the trial. *[J. Agric. Food Chem., 1998, 46 (1), pp 8–12]*

An interesting analysis from the University of Hong Kong showed that typical Cassia preps. have around 98% cinnamaldehyde and were effective against a wide range of pathogens, including Staphylococcus aureus, E. coli, Enterobacter aerogenes, Proteus vulgaris, Pseudomonas aeruginosa, Vibrio cholerae, Vibrio parahaemolyticus and Samonella. *[Am J Chin Med. 2006;34(3):511-22].*

Thyme

Thyme was used medicinally by the Egyptians, Greeks, and Romans. Most present day research has centered on thyme's ability as an antibacterial and anti-infectious agent, even when diffused in the air.

Thyme oil is composed of several different components that show antimicrobial activity (at least: carvacrol, thymol and linalool).

In vitro studies have shown that thyme oil has valuable broad spectrum activity against Salmonella typhimurium, Staphylococcus aureus, Escherichia coli, and a number of other bacterial species.

Thyme essential oils showed some of the strongest killing power against MRSA and VRE antibiotic-resistant bacteria, according to studies at the Western Infirmary, Glasgow, UK. According to Jean Valnet, M.D., thyme oil kills the anthrax bacillus, the typhoid bacillus, meningococcus, and the agent responsible for tuberculosis and is active against salmonella and staphylococcus bacteria.

The College of Pharmacy study at Oregon State University, also confirmed thyme is substantially more effective than most others in killing MRSA, including the virulent strain USA300. Oregano and thyme together are consistently the most effective in inhibiting the growth of all three bacteria; MRSA, Escherichia coli, and Acinetobacter calcoaceticus. Dr. Ihsan Edan AlSaimary, of the Univ. of Basrah, has also confirmed these other research results.

Thyme is also a broad spectrum disinfectant that helps to kill germs (including E.coli) on surfaces all around your home. *[Marino M, Bersani C, Comi, G. Antimicrobial Activity of the Essential Oils of Thymus vulgaris L. Measured Using a Bioimpedometric Method. Journal of Food Protection, Volume 62, Number 9, September 1999, pp. 1017-1023(7)].*

In another study, published in Bionews online, it was found that Escherichia coli and Salmonella typhimurium were susceptible to thymol and carvacrol (both found in thyme oil) and eugenol (found in clove oil).

Activity of natural antimicrobial compounds against Escherichia coli and Salmonella enterica serovar Typhimurium Letters in Applied Microbiology *[N.A. Olasupo, D.J. Fitzgerald, M.J. Gas-son and A. Narbad]* Volume 37 Issue 6 448 - December 2003

Thyme oil is very strong stuff by the way, don't go rubbing it on your skin without diluting it. Something like a massage oil.

Black Seed Oil

Black seed oil is not often included in Western reviews of essential oils. Maybe there is a certain amount of prejudice in this. But I think black seed oil could stand as high as Oregano oil and does not taste as repelling.

Black seed oil (Nigella sativa) has been known for centuries in Middle East countries. The black seed is known in Arabic as the habbutual barakah (the seed of blessing). It is sometimes called the Black Cumin Seed, however this is not the same as Black Cumin which the Indians refer to as Jeera/Zeera.

The Prophet Mohammad stated in his "Hadith" that black seed oil cures every illness except death. A small phial of it was apparently found in the tomb of Tutankhamen.

Now modern science has come to its support. Researchers around the world have confirmed the anti-bacterial and anti-mycotic effects of black seed oil. Health practitioners in various countries around the world are using the oil against inflamation of all sorts as well as fungi infections. Black Seed extracts have been found to stimulate bone marrow and immune cells, raise interferon production and increase B cells (which produce antibodies).

The active ingredients of black seed are nigellone, thymoquinone, and fixed oils. Beta si-tosterol has also been identified as a key marker in black seed oil. Beta sitosterol has been shown to exert protective effects and reduce symptoms of BPH (benign prostatic hyperplasia). *[Lancet 1995;345(8964):1529-32]*

Black seed also contains significant proportions of protein, carbohydrates and essential fatty acids. Other ingredients include linoleic acid, oleic acid, calcium, potassium, iron, zinc, magnesium, selenium, vitamin A, vitamin B, vitamin B2, niacin, and vitamin C.

Dose: a teaspoonful 3 times a day of the oil. It's bitter and irritating but can be mixed with tea, coffee, carrot juice, yoghurt or other carriers. For respiratory infections it can be rubbed in the chest; for sinusitis and catarrh, 3- 4 drops in each nostril.

General use: Ibn Senna known in the West as Avicenna (980-1037 AD) the Persian-born Islamic philosopher and physician who wrote the great medieval medical text, described the power of the black seed to stimulate the body's energy and banish fatigue.

A teaspoon of black seed oil mixed in a glass of orange juice with breakfast keeps you active all through the day. A teaspoon of black seed oil mixed in a hot drink after supper gives you a quiet sleep all through the night.

Mountain Savory

Long established as an antibiotic substitute, mountain savory (Satureja montana) was in third place, behind lemongrass oil and lemon mytle oil, according to a 2008 study *[Inhibition of methicillin-resistant Stapphulococcus aureus (MRSA) by essential oils; Sue Chao, Gary Young, Craig Oberg, and Karen Nakaoka; Flavour and Fragrance Journal, 2008; 23: 444-449]*.

One important study examined in vitro antimicrobial activity of the essential oils of the aerial parts of Satureja montana L. and Satureja cuneifolia. The major compound of S. montana oil was the phenolic monoterpene carvacrol (45.7%).

The antimicrobial effects of S. montana and S. cuneifolia oils were found to have a broad spectrum activity against multidrug-resistant pathogens. These oils were active against all the test strains, with the exception of Pseudomonas aeruginosa. Compared with S. cuneifolia, savory oil exhibited greater antimicrobial activity.

The maximum activity of savory oil was observed against Escherichia coli, MRSA and against the yeast (Candida albicans). The essential oil of S. cuneifolia was also found to inhibit the growth of medically important pathogens such as S. aureus and E. coli. Fungicidal activity for both oils against C. albicans and S. cerevisiae (food yeast) was also observed. *[Volume 18 Issue 12, s 967 – 970]*.

Useful antibiotic formula:

Mix together the following: 10 drops lemon; 8 drops mountain savory; 3 drops oregano; 1 tablespoon of V6 food grade oil. 2 ounces of grape juice.

Take 2 tablespoons a day of this mix. (based on a suggestion by Dr. Gary Young)

V6 is an essential oil carrier, consisting of fractionated Cocos Nucifera (Coconut) Oil, Sesamum Indicum (Sesame) Seed Oil, Vitis Vinifera (Grape) Seed Oil, Prunus Amygdalus Dulcis (Sweet Almond) Oil, Triticum Vulgare (Wheat) Germ Oil, Helianthus Annuus (Sunflower) Seed Oil, and Olea Europaea (Olive) Fruit Oil.

If you want, put it in a Double O gelatin or vegetable capsule instead of the V6. In which case use these proportions: 5 drops Lemon Essential oil 3 drops Oregeno Essential oil 5 drops Mountain Savory Essential oil

Take one capsule 3 times daily.

Pregnancy and Strep B

For pregnant women, Strep B can be a hazard (and to the neonate too). Signs, Symptoms of Neonatal GBS Infection Unaffected by Intrapartum Antibiotics *[Medscape Summary]*

"Antibiotic exposure also does not delay the onset of clinical signs of infection . . ."

[The Influence of Intrapartum Antibiotics on the Clinical Spectrum of Early-Onset Group B

Streptococcal Infection in Term Infants. Bromberger P, Lawrence JM, Braun D, Saunders B, Contreras R, Petitti DB, Pediatrics 2000 Aug;106(2):244-250]

In fact it probably causes it! [Potential consequences of widespread antepartal use of ampicillin. Towers CV, Carr MH, Padilla G, Asrat , Am J Obstet Gynecol 1998 Oct;179(4):879-83]

"The increased administration of antenatal ampicillin to pregnant women may be responsible for the increased incidence of early-onset neonatal sepsis with non-group B streptococcal organisms that are resistant to ampicillin. At this time penicillin G, rather than ampicillin, is therefore recommended for prophylaxis against group B streptococci. In addition, future studies are needed to determine whether alternate approaches, such as immunotherapy or vaginal washing, could be of benefit."

So, do the following:

Soak an ORGANIC tampon in 15 drops Lemon Essential oil 9 drops Oregeno Essential oil 15 drops Mountain Savory Essential oil 1 tsp carrier (V-6 food grade) oil Leave soaked tampon in overnight.

The Journal of the Science of Food and Agriculture Sep 2006 did a nice piece on growing savory (Satureja hortensis) in Scotland!) *[ref: S.G. Deans and K.P. Svoboda, Antibacterial activity of summer savory (Satureja hortensis L.) essential oil and its constituents. J. Hort. Sci., 64, 205-210 (1989)].*

Lavender

If you Google 101 essential oil uses, the first 23 are lavender!

Long prized for its healing properties, written records of the use of lavender for medicinal purposes date back as far as 60 AD and the writings of Dioscorides. In ancient Rome lavender was recognized for its healing and antiseptic qualities, its ability to deter insects, and for washing. In fact, its name stems from the Latin "lavare", meaning to wash. During the First World War, when modern antibiotics were sparse, lavender was used to dress wounds and helped to heal scar tissue and burns.

Lavender's Antibiotic Properties

Lavender is renowned for its antibiotic properties. Studies have shown that the essential oil of lavender, particularly when combined with Geranium oil, is capable of killing some Staph infections. Other studies have reported that lavender is good for treating ear infections, and is mild enough to treat such symptoms in children. Recently, four new chemicals have been isolated from lavender plants, and are believed to be beneficial for the treatment of Candida. Lavender tea (infusion) may be made from the dried flowers, 1 1/2 tsp. flowers to 8oz.water.

This can be drunk up to 4 times a day.

Lavender reduces fever and is a strong antiseptic and has been used to fight diphtheria, strep throat and pneumonia.

Lavender tea, or a few drops of oil in a glass of water, used as a gargle eases sore throats and laryngitis, can also soothe toothache.

Wounds and topical application

Lavender oil is an exception to all the other essential oils, in that it does not need to be diluted in a carrier oil because it is so gentle. It is also safe to use on infants and children.

Lavender is often used to treat scalds, minor burns, cuts, grazes, inflammation, eczema and dermatitis.

Geranium

This is Pelargonium sidoides, or South African Geranium NOT P. graveolens, the garden variety geranium. It's excellent for bronchitis. This is a big problem in primary care.

One study followed 476 adults with a clinical diagnosis of bronchitis from primary care medical centers in Germany. It excluded patients who had antibiotic therapy in the previous 4 weeks or asthma, severe heart, renal, or liver disease; immunosuppression; drug or alcohol abuse; and pregnancy or lactation.

This was a randomized, double-blind, placebo-controlled prospective study. Treatment consisted of 1.5 mL of aqueous ethanolic extract (11%) of Geranium root 3 times daily for 7 days. Placebo was matched for color, taste, smell, and viscosity. The breathlessness severity scale scores (BSS) improved in the geranium group over the placebo group. This was a well-structured trial.

[Matthys H, Eisebitt R, Seith B, Heger M. Efficacy and safety of an extract of Pelargonium sidoides (Eps 7630) in adults with acute bronchitis. A randomized, double-blind, placebo controlled trial. Phytomedicine 2003; 10(Suppl 4): S7-S17.]

Pelargonium is also an effective treatment for throat infections. Severe sore throat in children is often due to Streptococcus. In a double-blind clinical trial carried out in the Ukraine, children aged 6 to 10 with acute Strep throat infections were treated with pelargonium root extract or a placebo. Pelargonium resulted in much greater improvements than placebo, reduced the severity of symptoms and shortened the duration of illness by two days on average *[Altern Health Med 2003; 9(5): 68-79]*

Another study showed it was great for acute sinusitis, which is usually due to a bacterial or fungal infection after a cold. A recent study in Germany, involving 361 people with acute sinusitis who were treated with pelargonium root extract, found that at the end of the four week treatment period 80 per cent of patients recovered or experienced a clear improvement in their symptoms *[Z Phytother 2007; 28: 58-65]*.

One in vitro study showed killing drug-resistant Staph, so it may have a place in therapy for MRSA *[Phytomedicine 2003; 10 (Suppl 4): 18-24]*. The recommended dosage is 20mg of the root extract, three times a day, or 800mg of dried, powdered root, taken twice a day, for 10 days.

 General Warning: All I have written applies ONLY to therapeutic grade essential oils and not to recreational products, so please do not try some of its recommendation unless the oils you are using are at least AFNOR or ISO certified. Merely the word "pure" is not enough.

#40 Competitive Inhibition

In this section I'll be explaining another good strategy for controlling pathogenic bacteria. That's to encourage competition, so that safe, friendly organisms proliferate and occupy so much of the available territory (our bodies) that there is no room for wild forms to get started.

If the friendly horde that we carry should be replaced by nasty disease-causing renegade bacteria from the wild, our health can be compromised, even up to the point of death. All that really stops this happening is the massive presence of largely friendly—or at least nonhostile—forms. They are our main allies in fighting disease. Yet doctors ignore them and, indeed, even ravage and kill them in massive numbers, by the careless and unnecessary use of antibiotics.

Don't be smug. You do your part in hurting our friends too. Antiseptic soaps, sprays and body washes, that the TV ads convince you are really necessary, will kill off good forms as well as the ones you're scared of.

1. It's been said that we are landlords to the host of bacteria that live on us. As such, we should be responsible and caring owners and look after our guests! We can tend our crop of healthy organisms in several ways. We can feed the good bacteria.

2. We can import more good bacteria and add to them.

3. We can get other non-bacterial life forms to attack bacteria, much as introducing a new predator into the eco-landscape can result in wiping out the species on which it preys.

It may surprise you that the scientific study of these three strategies is well under way.

Adding to bacterial colonies is called "probiotics" and nurturing what's already present, with helpful nutrition, is called "pre-biotics".

Eubiotics, which covers both, means simply "good life"; in other words eating and drinking well and behaving sensibly. Synbiotics is another term you may encounter. I'll explain it further along.

The third approach we do using bacteria-hostile viruses which we call bacterio-phages; that means "bacteria eaters". We usually say phages for short. You can probably guess how that one works.

Next I'll cover each of these processes in more detail.

Probiotics

Probiotics, as I just remarked, means adding to the quantity of friendly organisms we carry. It is rather like artificially re-stocking lakes and rivers with fish. If you do it well—and actually ban fishing—you can build up stocks rapidly, because the fish will naturally reproduce and multiply. It's the same with helpful bacteria.

The first ever recognition of this process of probiotics was the use of yoghourt.

Russian scientist and Nobel laureate Eli Metchnikoff was the first to suggest that it would be possible to modify gut flora by adding friendly microbes to squeeze out the damaging ones.

At the beginning of the 20th century Metchnikoff, at that time a professor at the Pasteur Institute in Paris, introduced the theory that the aging process results from the activity of putrefactive (or proteolytic, meaning "breaks down protein") microbes producing toxic substances in the large bowel. According to Metchnikoff these compounds—including phenols, indols and ammonia—were responsible for what he called "intestinal auto-intoxication", which caused the physical changes associated with old age.

Metchnikoff knew that milk fermented with lactic-acid bacteria inhibits the growth of proteolytic bacteria because of the low pH (acidity) produced by the fermentation of lactose. He had also observed that certain rural populations in Europe, for example in Bulgaria and the Russian Steppes who lived largely on milk fermented by lactic-acid bacteria (yoghurt) were exceptionally long lived.

Based on these facts, Metchnikoff proposed that consumption of fermented milk would provide the intestine with harmless lactic-acid bacteria and decrease the intestinal pH and that this would suppress the growth of proteolytic bacteria (something else for the fans of alkali foods to think about).

Metchnikoff himself introduced in his diet sour milk fermented with the bacteria he called "Bulgarian Bacillus" and found his health benefited.

In 1900 Henry Tissier, also from the Pasteur Institute, isolated a Bifidobacterium. Tissier showed that bifidobacteria are predominant in the gut flora of breast-fed babies, and he recommended administration of bifidobacteria to infants suffering from diarrhea.

The stage then switched to Japan. In the 1920s Japan was not the wealthy nation it is today. Many children lost their lives to infectious diseases and other maladies brought on by malnutrition. In 1930. Dr. Minoru Shirota, working in a microbiology lab at Kyoto Imperial University's School of Medicine, succeeded in developing a stronger strain of lactic acid bacteria which would work to destroy the harmful gut bacteria. This bacterium was named Lactobacillus casei shirota after Shirota. It produced a yoghurt-like drink called Yakult, which was introduced to the market in 1935.

Subsequently, other species have been introduced to conventional medicine, including Lactobacillus rhamnosus, Lactobacillus casei, and Lactobacillus johnsonii, because they are normal intestinal species with beneficial properties.

Symbiotics

The old days of just "Lactobacillus acidophilus", basically a bovine form, are gone. As I said in my 1993 book, we need human strain Lactobacillus. The rest just don't thrive and soon die. Lactobacillus bulgaricus had the same problem.

But more importantly we need lots of Bifodobacteria, which is our main friendly passenger down there in the gut.

My more recent caution has been to get properly prepared organisms. The general technique of just crushing them into a tablet just kills the organisms, as you would expect, making a joke of the supposed population values given on the label.

Look instead for non-compacted preparations.

The other new trend is feeding your bowel flora the right stuff. No question that lots of yeasty foods to support the invaders, plus all the sugary and starchy foods that they can ferment for food, is a recipe for disaster. You need sugar-free healthy foods.

Keeping off ALL sugary and starch foods is tough. But you can take prebiotics, including galactooligosaccharides from human breast milk. Not for everybody but at least the conventional doctors have access to it. Mixing pre-biotics and probiotics like this is called synbiotics (syn- just means coming together, as in synthesize).

If you are not in a doctor's program for synbiotics, you need to consider rice bran and Inuflora, from the jerusalem artichoke. These are fiber products and provide a matrix in which the probiotics can establish themselves. One is soluble and one insoluble and the balance between the two makes an ideal, relatively inexpensive and natural substitute for fancy oligosaccharides.

There is the additional benefit of binding heavy metal complexes, when these are excreted into the gut via the hepato-biliary axis (liver and gallbladder excretion route).

Of course you probably know that holding yeasts, ferments and fungals in check is also a matter of avoiding dietary sugar, which feeds these organisms. Also the avoidance of all dietary fermented products will help, notably cheese, mushrooms, bread and so on.

So, you see, we've gone way beyond just adding yoghourt to our diets!

To summarize:

Bad foods (avoid):

- Yeasty, starchy, sugary, all artificial foods

- Limit fruits (sugar and fructose)

- Yoghourt preparations that have been sweetened for taste (rather defeats the purpose)

Good foods (eat plenty):

- Rice bran

- Inuflora. Jerusalem artichoke

- Any and all fiber vegetables, legumes and salad foods

If you Google "Inuflora" you will find scores of references and places where you can buy online.

This Is So Good The Veterinarians Are Onto It

Presenting his work at a Society for General Microbiology meeting in the UK on 2 April, 2009, Colin Hill of University College Cork described how his team had used three animal models of disease that had human counterparts — bovine mastitis, porcine salmonellosis (a gastrointestinal disease) and listeriosis in mice (an often fatal form of food poisoning) — to demonstrate the protective effects of probiotics.

The researchers used their own probiotic preparations containing safe bacteria such as Lactobacillus species newly isolated from human volunteers. Hill said that in all three animal diseases, the research group observed a positive effect, in that the animals were "significantly protected" against infection.

The team also used probiotics to control disease in animals that were already infected. The results of these tests, said Hill, showed that administering these safe bacteria to an infected animal was as effective as the best available antibiotic therapies in eliminating the infectious agent and resolving the symptoms.

In each instance the protection was linked to a particular bacterial species, and the mechanism of action varied from direct antagonism, where the probiotic directly kills the pathogenic bacteria, to effects mediated by the host immune system.

For example, Lactobacillus salivarius UCC118 protected mice against listeriosis (a disease which can affect pregnant women) by producing an antimicrobial peptide that eliminates Listeria monocytogenes, the causative organism of Listeria.

Probiotics directly help the effects of antibiotics!

It gets better!

Helicobacter pylori is present in about 25% of patients treated for gastritis or peptic ulcer disease (many now consider this microbe to be the "cause" of peptic ulcers). Standard treatment with two antibiotics (clarithromycin plus amoxicillin) and a fancy drug called a "proton pump inhibitor" (esomeprazole) failed to eradicate the troublesome microbe

But when a team from the University of Pisa in Italy added supplementation with probiotics (lactobacillus etc.), the cure rate was boosted and side effects reduced (less nausea, diarrhea, metallic taste in the mouth, inflamed tongue, and abdominal pain).

So now scientists think all 5 together are great.

You know what the joke is? If they just gave the probiotics they would work as well as or better than all the other drugs put together. And without any side effects. Duh!

[Am J Gastroenterol. 2007;102:951-956]

How To Take Probiotics

Forget the cheery TV ads with celebrity backing. Most commercial gut flora yoghurt products are of little value. They come with sugar! The bacteria are usually dead.

You need a good source of HUMAN strain lactobacillus. But also Bifidobacteria, which is normally the most common friendly organism in our gut, should be in the supplement as well.

Even then, the probiotic is not bound to establish itself successfully in our gut, so be very selective about what product you choose.

Beware of the tablet delivery. Most of those contain only crushed (dead) bacilli, no matter what claims of bacteria count! Capsules or liquid presentation are the safest.

Human Probiotic Therapy

(Faecal Transplants)

Are you ready for this? One of the ultimate ways to ehance bowel flora is to transplant faecal matter form healthy people into those who are sick and in danger.

Thye Yuck! factor is high but it does work and is practiced in many orthodox medical facilities around the world. In Sweden, human faecal transplants are the treatment of choice of life-threatening membranous ulcertaive colitis, a diosease typically caused by overuse and abuse of antibiotics, leading to overgrowth of Clostridium difficile. It is often fatal.

In fact the faeces are administered either via a nasogastric tube, straight into the stomach, or via an enema. The latter is surely to be preferred, since the colon is where these probiotic bacteria belong.

Of course there are precautions, like testing the "donor" for other pathogens and parasites, HIV and hepatitis.

Family members are preferred as donors, since we share about 80% of the bacteria colonists in the gut with our mother and siblings. But anyone can be a donor, provided he or she is healthy. Donors usually provide faecal material for free (well, you could hardly charge for it, come now!)

So what has all this to do with Clostridium difficile? This is a pretty toxic organism, as are most Clostridia species. But it's not native to our gut. It only takes hold when overuse of antibiotics have displaced the good guys. So it's a man-made complaint.

When healthy human gut flora is ploughed back, so to speak, C. difficile is squeezed out, exactly as we explain probiotics working. And before you ask: yoghourt won't work. This is a killer bug.

But faecal transplants seem to work very well indeed: close on 100% success in fact. People stretchered into hospital at death's door make a remarkable recovery, often in as little as 48 hours! That's amazing. It does suggest that the mechanism is specific toxins produced by friendly bacteria from a healthy gut being able to kill the C. difficile pretty quickly.

One study even resorted to my jokey approach and was titled: Bacteriotherapy using gut flora: toying with human motions" [Journal of Clinical Gastroenterology, vol. 38, p. 475].

However some 200 or so other studies were more serious.

One by Borody and colleagues details 6 cases of severe chronic ulcerative colitis treated using faecal bacteriotherapy. Complete reversal of symptoms was achieved in all patients in just 4 months, by which time all colitis medications had been discontinued as unnecessary [Borody T, Warren E, Leis S, Surace R, Ashman O (2003). "Treatment of ulcerative colitis using fecal bacteriotherapy.". J Clin Gastroenterol 37 (1): 42–7].

Bacteriophages

Phage – means eating in science. Esophag(e)us, the gullet, is the same word in a different form and phagocytes ("cell eaters") are immune cells that gobble up bacteria and viruses.

A bacteriophage is any one of a number of viruses that infect bacteria. Bacteriophages, or "phages" for short are viruses that invade only bacterial cells where they take over the genetic code and release more phages. When the bacterium dies, it releases these new phages and so they grow on and on. They can wipe out bacteria in no time.

Phages are estimated to be the most widely distributed and diverse entities in the biosphere. These ubiquitous organelles can be found in all reservoirs populated by bacterial hosts, such as soil or the intestines of animals. One of the densest natural sources for phages and other viruses is sea water and up to 70% of marine bacteria may be infected by phages.

You can find out more by visiting http://www.phage.org, which defaults to the Mansfield Ohio State University website.

A Historical Note

Following the discovery of bacteriophages by Frederick Twort and Felix d'Hérelle early in the 20th C, phage therapy was immediately recognized by many to be a key way forward for the eradication of bacterial infections.

Phages have since been used for over 60 years as an alternative to antibiotics in the former Soviet Union and Eastern Europe. In the USA during the 1940s, commercialization of phage therapy was undertaken by the large pharmaceutical company, Eli Lilly.

Whilst knowledge was being accumulated regarding the biology of phages and how to use phage cocktails correctly, early uses of phage therapy were often unreliable.

Unfortunately, when antibiotics were discovered and marketed widely in the USA and Europe, Western scientists mostly lost interest in further use and study of phage therapy for some time. But research continued in Russia and the Eastern Bloc.

I was taught about phages in med school in the early 1960s; then they seemed to disappear from view.

Phages are now making a comeback. They are seen as a possible therapy against multi drug resistant strains of many bacteria.

Pros and Cons Of Phage Therapy

There are some very important benefits with phage therapy. There are also some drawbacks.

Important benefits of phage therapy:

- Specific to the bacteria so it doesn't wipe out gut flora

- Harmless to the host

- Few side effects and do not stress the liver

- Only needs one dose because they replicate

Disadvantage:

• Will only kill the exact bacterium so needs a cocktail approach for multiple infections.

Biofilm, no not a Bond movie

Pseudomonas aeruginosa—which can cause a number of unpleasant and highly intractable infections, notably of the genito-urinary tract, but also ear infections—is particularly hard to treat because it typically wraps itself in a biofilm - a layer of sugars and proteins that make it up to 1000 times more resistant to antibiotics as a non-biofilm from the same species.

Now it has been found that a single dose of a phage called Biophage-PA, selectively attacks P. aeruginosa, breaks down the biofilm, and destroys the bacteria. It has been used successfully to treat long-term sufferers of antibiotic-resistant ear infections. Andrew Wright from University College London Ear Institute and colleagues studied 24 people with severe ear infections (Clinical Otolaryngology, accepted for publication). Half the volunteers were given Biophage-PA and the rest received a placebo.

Pain, pus secretion and inflammation were reduced in both groups, but the relief was double in the group on the treatment. The number of target bacteria in the ear was significantly reduced in the phage-treated group, while there was no significant reduction in the placebo group.

By the end of the six-week trial, three patients on the phage were clear of infection. Big promise there!

One of the important advantages of phage treatment is that it only takes one dose; this gets round the problem that patients often forget to complete their course of antibiotics, thus inviting resistance.

Of course it is entirely possible that bacteria might evolve resistance to phages too. It might almost be predicted. But so far it isn't documented.

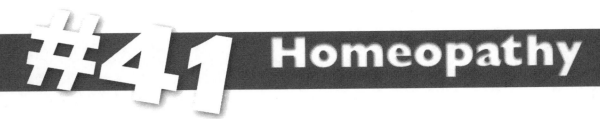

#41 Homeopathy

Now a New Science Altogether

Now, pay close attention, because this section will probably save more lives than any other in this report. I'm going to briefly describe homoeopathy, and explain why it is a wonderful, effective and safe approach to dealing with infections of all kinds (not just bacterial).

Homoeopathy has been around over two centuries, predates the vaccination and has demonstrated its effectiveness against countless infectious diseases and epidemics. In epidemics of the past, people who took homeopathy often survived unscathed, while others died in significant numbers. Yet, you will still hear it maligned and most conventional doctors and a pseudo-scientists claimed that it's been "proven not to work".

This is nonsensical logic. You cannot, logically and scientifically, prove something doesn't work! You can only fail to prove that it does work!

In fact detractors and bigots simply ignore the volumes of scientific evidence that homoeopathy works. Criticisms come from ignorant, mis-informed critics.

For example I always quote a major study reported in the prestigious journal The Lancet, [Lancet Dec 10, 1994:344, p 1585]. It caused a great deal of controversy and the then editor took the unusual step of mocking it in an editorial. But he did have the decency to admit the trials were done to a very vigorous standard (most drugs trials find their way to publications with far inferior standards).

Because he had to admit that using a double-blind randomized trial clearly showed that homeopathy worked, he wrote in his editorial:

"... we must ask if the technique of randomized controlled trials is fundamentally flawed, and capable of producing evidence for effects that do not exist, by, for example, the effects of clinicians' expectations of outcome transmitting by subtle effects that circumvent double blinding?" (Lancet 1994; 344;1601- 06) I regard this as the worst kind of bigotry. Instead of drawing the conclusion that homeopathy is indeed highly effective, he dared to suggest that randomized double-blind studies, the benchmark of medical science, maybe didn't really work!

Well, in reading this I know you are not too swayed by conventional rhetoric. Nevertheless, I urge that you do not permit this crass ignorance to enter your thinking. To go along with it could some day save your life.

If you trust your author, let me assure you that homeopathy works and it will save innumerable lives in a pandemic. As I indicated in an earlier section, I relied on it entirely when I lived in a malarious zone for 2 years. I took no prophylactic. I simply took a few doses of homeopathic anti-malaria preparation and then after a few weeks didn't even continue. I was bitten many times a day by mosquitoes but remained quite healthy.

Dana Ullman has done a great job of compiling lots of science papers showing uncontrovertibly that homeopathy does work. You can read her findings here:

http://www.homeopathic.com/articles/view,132 [DANA ULLMAN, MPH, is one of America's leading advocates for homeopathy. He has authored 10 books, including The Homeopathic Revolution: Why Famous People and Cultural Heroes Choose Homeopathy, Homeopathy A-Z, The Consumer's Guide to Homeopathy, Homeopathic Medicines for Children and Infants, Discovering Homeopathy, and (the best-selling) Everybody's Guide to Homeopathic Medicines, with co-author Stephen Cummings, MD].

Background

Homeopathy is a discipline developed during the 1790s entirely by one man: Samuel Hahnemann, a German physician. Experimenting on himself with the anti-malarial drug quinine, Hahnemann noticed that large doses of the medicine actually caused malaria-like symptoms, while smaller doses cured the symptoms. From this, he advanced his concept of Similia similibus curentur, or "let like be cured with like." Hahnemann then developed an extensive system of medicine based on this concept. He named it homeopathy, from the Greek words homoios (the same) and pathos (suffering).

As the homeopathic healing system grew in popularity during the 1800s, it quickly attracted vehement opposition from the medical and apothecary professions. Since the early 1900s, when the American Medical Association and pharmacists waged a battle against it, homeopathy has been neglected and sometimes ridiculed by mainstream medicine.

Proponents of homeopathy over the years have included Louisa May Alcott, Charles Dickens, Benjamin Disraeli, Johann Wolfgang Goethe, Nathaniel Hawthorne, William James, Henry Wadsworth Longfellow, Pope Pius X, John D. Rockefeller, Harriet Beecher Stowe, William Thackeray, Daniel Webster, and W. B. Yeats. England's royal family has employed homeopathic practitioners since the 1830s *[Source: About.com]*.

The only problem with this wonderful, gentle therapy, is that it takes some skill to administer. I hope, if there is a pandemic scare, or if you developed a drug-resistant strain of bacteria, you can get advice from someone properly trained.

Before you ask, Homeopathic Medicines are generally regarded as safe by the FDA (GRAS).

Homeopathy in 3 bullet points

Homeopathic remedies are almost always made from natural materials—plant, animal, or mineral substances or even venom from snakes or stinging insects. Some remedies may be given in a spray, ointment, or cream, but the most common forms of administration are liquid dilutions or dropped onto tablets or tiny pillules.

Here are the key points in how the preparations are made.

1. The key principle is "like treats like". A remedy which mimics the disease is chosen = similimum. This is the origin of the name "homo-" means: same as. It's completely different to the conventional idea of fighting and suppressing the symptoms

2. The remedy diluted many times: 10x10x10 (the X series, for example, 10X) or 100x100x100x100 etc (the C series eg. C30). Note that in Europe the X series is usually named D (for decimal), such as D8. Because this process makes the remedy work more effectively, it's called potentization.

3. After each dilution, the bottle is shaken or succussed as it's called.

The part that drives conventional thinkers crazy is the idea that diluting something makes it more effective. They "know" that diluting only makes it weaker. In fact they get very angry about the fact that most dilutions are so high that there cannot be even one single molecule of the original substance left in the remedy bottle.

But that's because they are bound by ridiculous constraints to their ideas and beliefs, which is that the only valid model is biochemical. In other words it needs "stuff" present to make it work.

The real nature of homeopathy seems to be acting as a signal to transfer a "message". This message can be passed onto the next solution and the next, no matter how many times the dilution process takes place.

I haven't time here to go into the whole science of homeopathy but let me offer you an illustration (overleaf), showing a spectrographic study of increasing dilutions of a remedy called belladonna. It should be a kind of "proof" to encourage you.

Read from the bottom up. The first solution is what we call the mother tincture (1:250). Each step in dilution, D1, D6, D12 and so on are progressive dilutions of this tincture, in the 10X sequence (decimal, hence D).

In this chart, any spikes above the horizontal line means that the belladonna solution is actually transmitting electro-magnetic energies (like radio or light waves). You will see that by D200 (diluting one drop to ten drops, repeated 200 times) the spikes are at their strongest.

I christened this chart "Radio Belladonna". What is remarkable is that the transmissions take place long after any of the belladonna substance has vanished.

Need I say more?

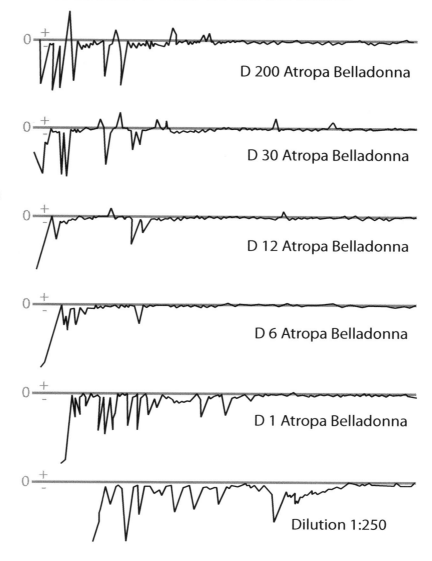

D 200 Atropa Belladonna

D 30 Atropa Belladonna

D 12 Atropa Belladonna

D 6 Atropa Belladonna

D 1 Atropa Belladonna

Dilution 1:250

Homoepathy In Acute Infections

Much homeopathy is directed towards lifting chronic or inherited disease traits. It requires what is called constitutional prescribing, meaning taking the persons whole physical make up and psychological character into the equation. Treatment is NEVER directed towards symptoms but towards changing the individual's make up or "constitution" and driving out disease tendency.

Prescribing for acute illnesses is rather different. Symptoms may be considered in their own right.

Homeopaths classify symptoms according to a hierarchy of four categories for purposes of acute prescribing:

• Peculiar symptoms. These are symptoms unique to the individual that do not occur in most persons with the acute disease. Homeopaths make note of peculiar symptoms because they often help to determine the remedy.

• Mental and emotional symptoms. These are important general symptoms that inform the homeopath about the patient's total experience of the disorder.

• Other general symptoms. These are physical symptoms felt throughout the patient's body, such as tiredness, changes in appetite, or restlessness.

• Particular symptoms. Particular symptoms are localized in the body; they include such symptoms as nausea, skin rashes, headache, etc.

During homeopathic case-taking, the practitioner will evaluate the intensity of the patient's symptoms, assess their depth within the patient's body, note any peculiar symptoms, evaluate the modalities of each symptom, and make a list of key symptoms to guide the selection of the proper medicine.

Medicines (called "remedies") can be general (against any infection) or specific for that disease.

General Remedies To Look Out For

Aconitum napellus: This remedy is often indicated when fever and inflammation come on suddenly, sometimes after exposure to wind and cold, or after a traumatic experience. The person may be very thirsty and often feels fearful or anxious.

Belladonna: Intense heat, redness, swelling, throbbing, and pulsation indicate a need for this remedy. The person's face may be flushed and hot (though hands and feet may be cold) and the eyes are often sensitive to light. Thirst may be lower than expected during fever. Discomfort is worse from motion or jarring, and relieved by cold applications. This was the classic remedy for scarlet fever.

Ferrum phosphoricum: This remedy is indicated in the early stages of many inflammations. Taken at the very first sign of a cold or sore throat, it often helps a person throw the infection off and not get ill. Fever, pink-flushed cheeks, a general weariness, thirst, and moderate pain and swelling are typical symptoms suggesting Ferrum phos in illness or infection.

Bryonia: Feeling worse from even the slightest motion is a strong indication for this remedy. When ill, the person wants to stay completely still—to be left alone and not interfered with in any way. Fever with chills, a very dry mouth, and thirst are also likely. Tearing pains that feel worse from any motion, but improve from pressure if it adds stability, may accompany local infections.

Calcarea carbonica: People who need this remedy tire easily and have low stamina. They tend to feel chilly and sluggish, with clammy hands and feet (though their feet may heat up in bed at night, and their heads may perspire during sleep). Swollen lymph nodes, frequent colds, sore throats, ear infections, and skin eruptions are common. Children who need this remedy are often slow to walk and may have teething problems, frequent colds, and ear infections.

Hepar sulphuris calcareum: A person who needs this remedy feels extremely sensitive and vulnerable when ill, especially if exposed to cold or drafts. Ear infections, sore throats, sinusitis, bronchitis, and skin eruptions are often seen, and cheesy-smelling discharge or offensive pus may be produced. Areas of inflammation can be very sore and sensitive, and splinter-like pains are often felt (in the tonsils when swallowing, in a boil when the skin is touched, etc.).

Silica: A person who needs this remedy can be sensitive and nervous, with low stamina and poor resistance to infection—leading to swollen lymph nodes, frequent colds, sore throats, tonsillitis, sinusitis, bronchitis, and other illnesses. Boils, easy infection of wounds, and abscessed teeth are often seen. Although very chilly in general, the person often perspires during sleep. Offensive foot sweat with an inclination toward fungal infections is also common.

Mercurius solubilis: This remedy is needed when a person has swollen lymph nodes, offensive breath, and is extremely sensitive to any change in temperature. A tendency toward night sweats and profuse salivation during sleep are other indications. Infections of the gums, ears, sinuses, throat, and skin often respond to this remedy when the other symptoms fit.

Sulphur: This remedy is useful in many kinds of infection characterized by irritation, burning pain, redness of mucous membranes, and offensive odors and discharges. Skin problems are very common—eczema, acne, boils, lymphangitis, and inflammations on or around the genitals. Symptoms are often worse from warmth and worse after bathing. Colds, bronchitis, and other illnesses that have been neglected, or infections that drag on for a very long time, may be helped with this remedy

Specific Remedies Or Nosodes

Another approach entirely is to use disease pathogen of diseased tissues as a remedy. Remember, it will be diluted many times and so quite harmless. So hoemopathically-potentized malaria can be used as an anti-malaria remedy and that's what I referred to earlier. I took it in Sri Lanka.

The use of actual disease substances we call a "nosode". Nosodes exist for TB, cancer, rubella, 'flu, Streptococcus and Staphylococcus, to name just a few.

A nosode can act like a vaccine and be used as a preventative. In fact Samuel Hahnemann should be credited with the development of vaccination, not Edward Jenner (but try telling that to orthodox doctors!)

Nosodes are really only available through a homeopathic prescriber. In the event of an epidemic or pandemic, I expect supplies will be limited.

But if you are OK ordering online, you can get ANYTHING homeopathic from India, where homeopathy is huge. That's thanks to the former ruler of Punjab, Maharaja Ranjit SinghMaharaja, who espoused it in 1830. It worked for him and he spent some of his fabulous fortune disseminating it throughout India (which included Pakistan at that time).

Every major city in India has pharmacies dispensing homeopathy medicine. Many states in India also have homeopathy colleges teaching this type of alternative medicine to prospective students. Currently there are 186 homeopathic medical colleges in India.

The Indian government created the Central Council Of Homeopathy which requires uniform education at the graduate level and diploma level in homeopathy. This has lead to standardized practice in India preventing unqualified homeopaths to prescribe medicine and treatments. Currently, there are over 300,000 homeopathic doctors practicing medicine in India.

Just to finish, if you have not heard the term "allopathic", it means conventional medicine. It comes from the Latin alli- meaning "other" (same word as AL-ternative). So it's the direct opposite of treating like with like. Allopathic medicine fights against a condition, trying to suppress it, rather than working along with it, to bring it to a close.

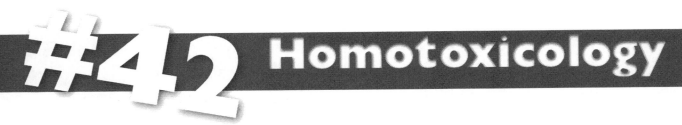

#42 Homotoxicology

Also know as comlex homeopathy and German homeopathy.

A similar and closely related discipline is that of homotoxicology, sometimes called "complex homeopathy". It's also sometimes called "German homeopathy", since around 40% of German MDs use it regularly. But I think that's confusing, because Hahnemann was German so both methods are really "German homeopathy".

Complex doesn't really mean convoluted and difficult; it means by the use of mixtures and formuals, instead of single pure substances.

In fact complex homeopathy, as it is practiced today, was largely developed by another German doctor Hans-Heinrich Reckweg. He sold out his company in Baden-Baden and re-started in Albuqueque, New Mexico, so you have it in the US too. It's called HEEL (short for herba est ex luce, or plants are from light).

Complex homeopathy, as its name suggests, uses compound solutions; mixes of different remedies. This is anathema to classic homeopaths, who insist that Hahnemann described a science based on one remedy, one disease, at one time (they just ignore the fact that even Hahnemann later experimented with mixes.

Different formulations

Because of the very nature of homeopathy, mixtures can take two forms: mixtures of different substances or mixtures of the same substance only but at different potencies or dilutions. The latter we call a chord (like in music, several notes sounding at once).

But there are other, more subtle differences too. In complex homeopathy we tend to use lower (not so extreme) dilutions. Thus D4, D6 and D10 are often encountered; D30, D60 and D200 are also encountered a lot. Whereas a classic homeopath works more in dilutions (potencies) of C12 and upwards to 1M and 2M. M means a 1:100 dilution, repeated 1,000 times.

In classical homeopathy, the teaching is that as soon as you get a result, you stop the medication and leave the recovery process to run un-aided. A complex homeopathy prescriber would tend to smile with satisfaction and write the patient up for another week or two! Then, as well as the scandal of using more than one substance at a time in a mixture, a complex homeopathy prescriber might also use more than one mixture at a time!

This is typical where we would add what's called a "drainage remedy". This is to increase removal of toxins which accrue in an illness, especially when being treated effectively. As the pathogens are destroyed, the body may reach an overload state, due to its inability to remove resulting toxins fast enough. Drainage remedies stimulate that process and so make sense.

Here an example of a complex homeopathic remedy (Lymphomyosot) and what it contains and simplified notes on what each is for:

Geranium robertianum 4X, diarrhea, painful urination, ulcerations Nasturtium aquaticum (watercress) 4X, liver and gall bladder, mouth ulcers Ferrum iodatum 12X, scrofula (TB), glandular swelling Myosotis arvensis 3X, chronic bronchitis

Scrophularia nodosa (knotted figwort) 3X, inflammation and swelling of lymph glands and breast, eczema Teucrium scorodonia (germander) 3X, chronic rhinitis, bronchitis, tuberculosis

Veronica officinalis (speedwell) 3X, chronic bronchitis, cystitis, dermatosis

Equisetum hyemale (horsetail) 4X, cystitis, kidney stones

Fumaria officinalis (fumitory) 4X, blood purifier, excess toxin levels

Natrium sulphuricum 4X, liver problems, gastroenteritis, asthma Pinus sylvestris (Scots pine) 4X, rickets, bronchitis, scrofula

Gentiana lutea (yellow gentian) 5X, chronic gastritis, flatulence and diarrhea.

Aranea diadema (spider orchid) 6X, exudations, worse in wet and cold

Sarsaparilla 6X, herpes, painful urination, cystitis and kidney inflammation

Calcarea phosphorica 12X, gastroenteritis, rickets

Note some similarities with herbal preparations.

What To Take

Complex homoepathy prescribing is a complex art in itself. I cannot do more than give an outline here. However it's definitely the one for home prescribing. There are four main reason why it is good for the layman to use:

1. It's safe, you can't mess up.

2. Reactions are milder, it's hard to overdo it!

3. The very nature of a mixture means something should hit the target!

4. The names often help with knowing what to choose (no such help in classic homeopathy)

Here are some suggestions what to do for a severe infection.

Engystol N (HEEL). Great for boosting defence mechanisms and increasing resistance to infections of all kinds, especially viral infections. Good for pneumonia, bronchitis, rhinitis and hepatitis. It's also good after vaccinations, to prevent adverse after effects.

Echinacea compositum

I have already remarked I wouldn't put much faith in just Echincaea for my family. But this Echinacea compositum (complex) is brilliant!

Euphorbium Compositum Spray

Great for nasal, sinus and pharygeal infections.

Galium-Heel is a non-specific drainage remedy, perhaps more suitable for chronic conditions.

Gripp-Heel. This is the one you want in a swine flu or bird flu pandemic. Grippe is the French word for influenza. It contains Aconite (shock and chills, which is the onset of most infectious diseases); Bryonia (inflammation of mucus membranes and cough); Lachesis (bushmaster snake), worsening condition and congestive bronchitis; Eupatorium, influenza with excruciating pains; and Phosphorus, bronchopneumonia and laryngitis, with hoarseness.

Lymphomyosot. Chronic and repeated tonsillitis and lymph gland swellings.

Tonsilla compositum. This is one of my favorites for stimulating the immune system. It has no less than 29 logical ingredients and increases body defences in all ways, but especially the lymphatic system. It goes to chills, bronchitis, emphysema, abcesses, suppurating wounds, gingivitis, as well as the obvious sore throats and tonsillitis.

There are many other compounds which can be called into action by the experienced and knowledgeable prescriber. It takes years to learn the full repertoire for this kind of prescribing.

But here is information enough to get you started on searching and, hopefully, to give you confidence that here is a wonderful, safe and gentle approach to healing. No matter how it is mocked and despised by conventional colleagues who only prescribe poisonous drugs as a "cure", trust me, complex homeopathy works!

Where To Buy

HEEL have distributors and outlets in many parts for the world, from Colombia to Bielorus! For the UK and several other centers, contact my good friend Roger Wilson via his website, http://www.biopathica.co.uk (or biopathica.com).

HEEL's headquarters are in Germany: Dr.-Reckeweg-Str. 2-4 D-76532 Baden-Baden or

P.O. Box 100349 D-76484 Baden-Baden Phone: +49 72 21 50 10 0 E-Mail: info@heel.de Web: http://www.heel.de

HEEL USA (www.heelusa.com) is related by the Reckeweg range of products but is a separate corporate entity to the original HEEL.

There are several other very good complex homeopathic pharmacy suppliers:

Deseret Biologicals in Sandy, Utah.

Deseret Biologicals are now working with Bruce Shelton MD, former US advisor to HEEL. 469 West Parkland Drive Sandy, UT 84070-6403

phone: 801-563-7448 fax: 801-563-7455 orders: 800-827-9529

Pascoe. Not so much for otc remedies or direct mail but you will recognize these products from certain prescribers. [http://www.pascoe-global.com/sites/content/e7639/e16201/index_ eng.html]

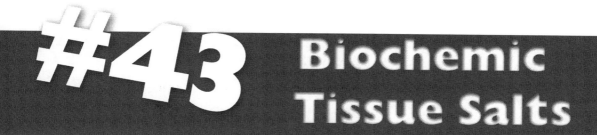

#43 Biochemic Tissue Salts

Also known as Schussler Salts

Biochemic tissue salts were developed as homeopathic remedies by Samuel Hahnemann, and further investigated by Dr Wilhelm Heinrich Schuessler in the late nineteenth century. They are remedies based on the inorganic salts and are intended to increase the body's ability to absorb and use the mineral salts found in a person's everyday diet in order to maintain or restore good health.

According to Schuessler, illnesses arise when there is an imbalance or deficiency of these minerals in the body - when they are not in the right place at the right time, in other words. Schuessler salts, which he called 'means of functioning,' are meant to redress the imbalance. Schuessler himself worked with 12 salts. His successors added 12 more.

Modern Tablet Form

Biochemic tissue salts are available in tablet form similar to that of most homeopathic remedies. They are made up of the salt ground with lactose powder (a process called trituration) in a ratio of 1:9, and then further diluted six times at a 1:9 ratio so the final product is a 1,000,000 to 1 dilution. These tablets then dissolve on the tongue. They are both individually available as one kind of salt, or come in combinations to address particular illnesses or ailments. There are no known side-effects, and taking them in excess will not result in overdose as biochemic tissue salts occur naturally in the body. Waste will be excreted.

We don't need all the Schuessler salts here but two are useful for infections:

Ferrum Phosphate (ferrum phos) D12 or 12X: great for acute infections, the quicker you nip them in the bud, the better.

Kali Muriaticum/ Potassium Chloride (kali mur) D6 or 6X: the second good infection remedy, can be taken alternately with Ferr Phos.

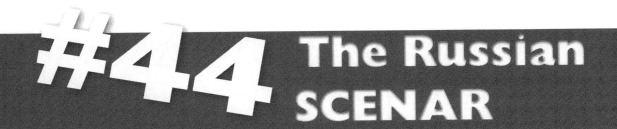

#44 The Russian SCENAR

I strongly recommend every home have a SCENAR in the medicine cabinet. I have seen this amazing device blow away serious infections in a day or less.

Actually, the SCENAR is a whole family of machines developed in Russia and I predict they will completely change the face of medicine in the next 20 years. They are fast, portable, cheap and effective against almost any condition, from treating sports injuries, strokes, angina, acute infections, back pains and irritable bowel disease (as well as pre-menstrual tension and post-surgical complications) and even defibrillating hearts!

The promise of a small hand-held device that is capable of curing most illness, such as was portrayed in the cult 1970s TV series "STAR TREK", has become a reality. The device weighs around 300 gm, resembles a TV remote control and is powered by an ordinary 9v. battery. It is placed on the skin of the chest, head, abdomen or any diseased part, where it collects electromagnetic signals. These are then modulated according to the on-board software programme and played back to the tissues.

Essentially, SCENAR is using the patient's own endogenous signals on a cybernetic feedback basis, scanning and re-transmitting many times a second. As described to me, the device 'evolves' a new signal pattern for the disordered tissues, the machine literally entering into an information dialogue with the body. New frequencies and energy patterns are established, which in turn become fresh input signals, to be further modified, and so on.

This output-equals-new- input is much the way that fractals are generated and thus, biologically-speaking, we seem to be on good ground here. On the premise that disease signals are generally fixed and unnatural, anything which breaks up the existing order has the capability of disease-busting.

SCENAR casebook from Dr Keith MD (quoted in my book "Virtual Medicine").

Male, 69 years old. This man who was a gardener by profession had chronic suppurating osteomyelitis of the foot (deep bone infection) which could not be controlled. He was scheduled for an amputation of the lower leg in four days time, largely due to intractable pain. Someone decided to try a SCENAR device on him. It was run over the affected limb for about 30 minutes. Next day, the pain had vanished for the first time in 8 months. Later that day another 30-minute treatment was given.

By next morning the recovery was so dramatic the amputation was called off. A third treatment was given and seven days after the first SCENAR this man was back at work, digging in the garden. His leg has completely recovered.

Clinical Aspects

The device is very safe; the impulse times are very short. No pain is felt but the patient is usually aware of a tingling sensation while it works. The practitioner seeks for what the Russians term asymmetry, meaning something different about the tissue characteristics in the vicinity. There are five main criteria: discolouration (reddening or pallor) sensation (numbness or hyper-aesthesia) stickiness' in which the machine drags with a magnet-like quality as it is drawn over certain tracts of the skin sound changes (the machine begins to chatter electronically as it hits certain zones) change in numerical output display.

Even though it may not coincide with the obvious area of symptoms or pathology, the important point is to treat the asymmetry. For reasons we do not fully understand, when this is eliminated, recovery will rapidly follow.

Couldn't resist reporting just a simple application... My lovely wife Vivien was working in Los Angeles (she's a fashion designer). She had a respiratory infection and felt rough enough for antibiotics. However she was still suffering when she came home Friday night. I broke out the SCENAR and ran it over her chest and back. Within 5 minutes there was what the Russians called an "asymmetry": on the left side there was pain under the tip of the scapula and over the pecs at the front. We worked this for about 10 minutes.

That's all! She reported feeling tons better. All night she didn't cough and woke feeling much better. Who needs antibiotics or even herbs and homeopathy when you have a SCENAR!

You can find out more about this device in my book "Virtual Medicine". Get it here:

http://www.alternative-doctor.com/scenar/

#45 UV Light As An Antibiotic

Back when (in the days before antibiotics) there were many treatments which worked for infections. One almost lost technique was the use of Ultra Violet Light irradiation of the blood to kill pathogens and even cancer cells.

This is a version of what we technically call plasmapheresis or, in Europe "auto sanguis" therapy (meaning "own blood" therapy).

You can do a number of things to blood while it is outside the body that you could not do while it is inside... For example, you can expose it to ozone and so enrich it with oxygen. A high local concentration of oxygen is known to provide a hostile environment for cancer cells. Some deadly organisms, too, like the gas gangrene bacteria (Clostridium welchii), are killed by a high-oxygen environment. Even viruses succumb.

But here I am describing the use of ultra-violet light to treat infections. UV is accepted as a sterilizing agent; city water supply is treated with it; indeed, you may have a UV unit fitted to your spa or pool. There is no scientific argument over its cleansing capabilities. It zaps pathogens!

It's toxic to humans too (sunburn!) but that problem is solved by focusing the UV on blood which is OUTSIDE the body. We call this ultra-violet blood irradiation or UVBI for short. It's also sometimes known as photoluminescence.

The treated blood is returned to the body, where it spreads its good message throughout the tissues. Surprisingly, only about 5% of the total blood volume needs to be treated in this way. This small proportion spreads through the entire body and works its magic, in much the same way a therapeutic drug gets everywhere.

UVBI kills viruses, parasites and bacteria and was popular in the 1930s for polio and other viral infections. The reason is simple enough: it works! But then it became unpopular, as it was gradually sidelined by mass vaccination programs, which were believed to work, despite evidence to the contrary. Finally, UV blood therapy fell into disrepute, except among dedicated holistic physicians.

That's a great pity because it is very safe (no side effects ever recorded, when used properly), highly effective and cheap to do. It's so easy, as a matter of fact, that it's something a lay persons, with the right equipment and clear instructions, can administer it to themselves.

History

Research into the use of UV light for therapy goes back as far as the 1870's. Niels Ryberg Finsen won the Nobel Peace Prize for "Physiology of Medicine" in 1903 for his UV treatments of 300 people suffering from Lupus in Denmark.

One of the early pioneers of UVBI was Kurt Naswitis, who directly irradiated the blood with UV light through a shunt in 1922.

Another pioneer of this treatment was Emmett K. Knott, who started up in 1928. Dr. Virgil K.

Hancock and Mr. Knott published the first article on the therapeutic efficacy of phototherapy in June of 1934. By June of 1942 they had treated 6,520 patients with ultraviolet therapy. Their work was reported in the most prestigious medical journals. One respected physician of the time, Dr. Rebbeck, wrote in the early 1940s that Hancock and Knott "had in the irradiation of blood with ultraviolet spectral energy, a therapy of more pronounced value than any other method known to date." During a 50-year period, doctors performed more than 300,000 clinical tests that repeatedly showed photoluminescence works and not a single patient was harmed.

Factually, there are very few contraindications for UVBI and unsuitable patients are easily screened out: porphyria, hereditary metabolic disorders such as phenylketonuria, exeroderma pigmentosum, acute photodermatitis, and a hypersensitivity to sunlight or other forms of ultraviolet light are not suitable for UVBI.

On September 11, 1928 Emmet K. Knott patented his device as a "Means for Treating Bloodstream Infections" and later he received another patent, in 1943, which was slightly different.

This is very fortunate for us today because the machine received an FDA "grandfather" status as a device that was sold and distributed in interstate commerce prior to 1976.

Procedure

If you are lucky enough to locate a practitioner who will do this for you, you will find it's very quick and virtually painless. It takes about 20 minutes in total.

A catheter is placed into one of the veins around the elbow (usually with a butterfly needle -- a small plastic catheter attached to a short needle). Drawn blood travels through a small glass chamber, called a cuvette, where it is exposed twice to ultraviolet light before getting re-introduced to the patient's blood stream.

Many patients feel significant improvements after just a few treatments. In severe cases, patients may require 10 or more treatments. But usually, 3 to 5 treatments are sufficient. Even chronic, intractable problems will likely recover.

What Conditions Can Be Benefited?

Actually, a knowledgeable practitioner would probably say almost any non-optimum condition might respond, even cancer. Bear in mind my rubric that "Any good health measure is an anti-cancer measure."

Other conditions which may be significantly improved include:
- Viral Infections
- Candidiasis (fungal infections)
- Bacterial Infections
- Chronic Fatigue
- Poor Oxygen
- Blood Poisoning
- Chronic infections (skin, etc.)
- Colitis
- Leg ulcers
- Diabetes Complications
- Poor Immune Function

UVBI or photoluminescence seems poised to make a come back. It is free of (legal) molestation by the FDA, though the FDA has scant regard for the niceties of law!

But with the obvious dangers and lack of efficacy of vaccination; the development of dangerous antibiotic resistant species of bacteria; and with the difficulty eradicating many viruses, such as hepatitis and AIDS, it is good to know we have a PROVEN, safe, fast, cheap and effective alternative therapy. It won't suit the mindless pill-pushers, who seem to have lost the true art of the healer.

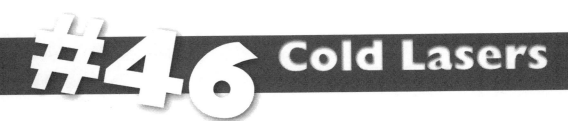

#46 Cold Lasers

The local application of low-level laser (cold laser) energy has been found to be effective in a variety of inflammatory conditions, including infections. Lasers produce coherent light, which is critical. Color light therapy is a different topic altogether. LED light sources are non-coherent.

The 630- 640 nanometre wavelength (red) has considerable effect on the tissues, stimulating cell metabolism, decreasing inflammation and increasing endorphin release, which reduces pain.

One other important consideration is the optimum power necessary for bio-stimulation. The Arndt-Schulz Law of photo-biological activity, essentially states that "less is more" when it comes to energy for improved cellular physiology. A good cold laser, such as the Erchonia cold laser provides the best wavelength (635 nm) for cellular physiology at very low energy (2-5 mill Watts) to stimulate cells to function better. If the stimulation is too intense, there may actually be an inhibitory effect, or possibly degeneration or destruction of cells.

The advantage of lasers, like the SCENAR is that they can be focused on the area of concern. There is no local thermal effect and no recovery time. Normal healing requires certain mediators to be released at the wound site. These cell mediators call inflammatory cells to the wound which clean up damaged tissues, fight bacteria, and stimulate specialized cells to grow to try to heal the zone of injury. The physiologic concept is that cold laser improves cellular metabolism and accelerates the process of healing to a more rapid and efficient state.

Now it happens that 405 nm (violet) laser light works differently. It is soothing and calming.

It helps the body fight infections at a deeper level and even seems to bring in an emotional response to healing.

Stress, overwork, improper diet and the environment can all contribute to a toxic overload in the body which reduces the body's ability to maintain a healthy immune system. The immune system is the body's defense against viruses, bacteria, molds, fungus and other opportunistic infections which would like to set up a "home" in your body. The laser can help detoxification protocols work faster and on a deeper cellular level.

There are over 1500 published studies and not one of them mentions any negative side effects of semi-conductor diode lasers at the 5mW range, such as the Erchonia lasers. Cold lasers are safe, non-toxic and non-invasive - there have not been any recorded side effects in over 1500 publications. There are some necessary common sense precautions that need to be considered, such as avoiding pointing the laser beam directly into the eye and maintaining it there, which could prove to be damaging to the eye.

Note: If you hear the term "scalar wave laser" run a mile. There is no such thing in the universe and it's science baloney. Find a real science-grounded practitioner, not someone who speaks pseudo-quantum psychobabble.

#47 Nano UV Zapper

This is another device which should be in every home. Manufacturers claim it is the "world's first compact disinfection light" and say the technology could be used for germ-busting in homes, schools and hospitals.

The Nano-UV Portable Disinfection Light looks like a mobile phone but flips open to reveal an ultraviolet lamp.

Those behind the product say it is certified to kill 99.99 per cent of the potentially deadly H5N1 strain of avian flu in five seconds, and harmful bacteria, such as MRSA, E.coli and salmonella, in 10 seconds.

By using "multi-wavelength" UV technology, combining UVA, UVB and UVC rays, manufacturers say the light is more effective than standard UV disinfection products at killing the DNA of viruses, bacteria and fungi.

The light has a sterilising effect when passed over objects like baby's dummies, nappy changing tables, cutlery, toilet seats and towels.

The Nano UV zapper has a built-in safety device to ensure each use only lasts 10 seconds, which is all it takes to kill 99% plus of all germs.

The beauty of this product is that it's small enough to carry everywhere and powerful enough to give you peace of mind in any situation.

The Nano zapper can be used to sterilize any surface except the skin.

Microbiologist Professor Hugh Pennington, the emeritus professor of bacteriology at Aberdeen University, said UV technology is well known for its germ-killing properties and has a place alongside other good hygiene practices, such as hand-washing.

#48 What Goes In The Medicine Cupboard?

Let's finish up by considering what should every home have in the medicine cupboard. Having got this far, you may have your own opinions about what would be good to include, to be ready in the event of an infection, whether mild or severe.

These are the items I suggest:

- 1 oz. or 25 grams of icthammol ointment (20%)

- Drawing salve for acute, small inflamed infections

- 4 oz. spray of colloidal silver; 100 ml. bottle Grazes, skin abrasions, dental hygiene, sore throat, puncture wounds

- A bottle of MMS (chlorine dixiode) Severe systemic infections, viral and bacterial, bronchitis, wounds, abcesses

- Engystol (if you can't get it, use propolis) General defence for any infectious disease, especially viral.

- 30 ml. bottle of Samento (TOA-free) Chronic infections and "stealth pathogens" (eg. Lyme's)

- 30 ml. Oregano Oil Acute infections of all kinds

- 30 ml. Black seed oil Acute infections of all kinds

- 30 ml. Lavender Oil Mainly skin conditions but could be used for abscesses, acne, athlete's foot, fungal infections, boils, bruises, cuts, insect bites and stings, lice, sunburns, wounds, bronchitis, coughs, colds, congestion, flu, laryngitis, throat infections, whooping cough, and sinus infections.

- Also You Need One Of Two Electrical Healing Devices.

    A SCENAR

    Learn to use it first; don't wait till somebody gets sick!

A low-level laser

Also learn to use it first!

- High Dose Vit C and Vit A for acute viral infections. Have vitamin C powder on hand and vitamin A capsules. There are 25,000 IU capsules coming in from China. Buy them only if you trust the source (I don't).

- Vitamin D capsules, 5,000 IU, improve your immunity whenever an epidemic threatens

Appendix

I thought you might like to supplement what I am telling you with the "official" story. This section is from the FDA Consumer magazine (September 1995). I think it's worth reading it over again in a different way. It re-inforces what I have been saying.

You can also listen to some useful recordings and download PDF files here too:

When penicillin became widely available during the Second World War, it was a medical miracle, rapidly vanquishing the biggest wartime killer--infected wounds.

Discovered initially by a French medical student, Ernest Duchesne, in 1896, and then rediscovered by Scottish physician Alexander Fleming in 1928, the product of the soil mold Penicillium crippled many types of disease-causing bacteria. But just four years after drug companies began mass-producing penicillin in 1943, microbes began appearing that could resist it.

The first bug to battle penicillin was Staphylococcus aureus. This bacterium is often a harmless passenger in the human body, but it can cause illness, such as pneumonia or toxic shock syndrome, when it overgrows or produces a toxin.

In 1967, another type of penicillin-resistant pneumonia, caused by Streptococcus pneumoniae and called pneumococcus, surfaced in a remote village in Papua New Guinea. At about the same time, American military personnel in Southeast Asia were acquiring penicillin-resistant gonorrhea from prostitutes.

By 1976, when the soldiers had come home, they brought the new strain of gonorrhea with them, and physicians had to find new drugs to treat it. In 1983, a hospital-acquired intestinal infection caused by the bacterium Enterococcus faecium joined the list of bugs that outwit penicillin.

Antibiotic resistance spreads fast. Between 1979 and 1987, for example, only 0.02 percent of pneumococcus strains infecting a large number of patients surveyed by the national Centers for Disease Control and Prevention were penicillin-resistant. CDC's survey included 13 hospitals in 12 states. Today, 6.6 percent of pneumococcus strains are resistant, according to a re-port in the June 15, 1994, Journal of the American Medical Association by Robert F.

Breiman, M.D., and colleagues at CDC. The agency also reports that in 1992, 13,300 hospital patients died of bacterial infections that were resistant to antibiotic treatment.

Why has this happened?

"There was complacency in the 1980s. The perception was that we had licked the bacterial infection problem. Drug companies weren't working on new agents. They were concentrating on other areas, such as viral infections," says Michael Blum, M.D., medical officer in the Food and Drug Administration's division of anti-infective drug products. "In the meantime, resistance increased to a number of commonly used antibiotics, possibly related to overuse of antibiotics. In the 1990s, we've come to a point for certain infections that we don't have [antibiotics] agents available."

According to a report in the April 28, 1994, New England Journal of Medicine, researchers have identified bacteria in patient samples that resist all currently available antibiotic drugs.

Survival of the Fittest

The increased prevalence of antibiotic resistance is an outcome of evolution. Any population of organisms, bacteria included, naturally includes variants with unusual traits--in this case, the ability to withstand an antibiotic's attack on a microbe. When a person takes an antibiotic, the drug kills the defenseless bacteria, leaving behind--or "selecting," in biological terms--those that can resist it. These renegade bacteria then multi-ply, increasing their numbers a millionfold in a day, becoming the predominant microorganism.

The antibiotic does not technically cause the resistance, but allows it to happen by creating a situation where an already existing variant can flourish. "Whenever antibiotics are used, there is selective pressure for resistance to occur. It builds upon itself. More and more organisms develop resistance to more and more drugs," says Joe Cranston, Ph.D., director of the department of drug policy and standards at the American Medical Association in Chicago.

A patient can develop a drug-resistant infection either by contracting a resistant bug to begin with, or by having a resistant microbe emerge in the body once antibiotic treatment begins. Drug-resistant infections increase risk of death, and are often associated with prolonged hospital stays, and sometimes complications. These might necessitate removing part of a ravaged lung, or replacing a damaged heart valve.

Bacterial Weaponry

Disease-causing microbes thwart antibiotics by interfering with their mechanism of action. For example, penicillin kills bacteria by attaching to their cell walls, then destroying a key part of the wall. The wall falls apart, and the bacterium dies. Resistant microbes, however, either alter their cell walls so penicillin can't bind or produce enzymes that dismantle the antibiotic.

In another scenario, erythromycin attacks ribosomes, structures within a cell that enable it to make proteins. Resistant bacteria have slightly altered ribosomes to which the drug cannot bind. The ribosomal route is also how bacteria become resistant to the antibiotics tetracycline, streptomycin and gentamicin.

How Antibiotic Resistance Happens

Antibiotic resistance results from gene action. Bacteria acquire genes conferring resistance in any of three ways.

In spontaneous DNA mutation, bacterial DNA (genetic material) may mutate (change) spontaneously (indicated by starburst). Drug-resistant tuberculosis arises this way.

In a form of microbial sex called transformation, one bacterium may take up DNA from another bacterium. Pencillin-resistant gonorrhea results from transformation.

Most frightening, however, is resistance acquired from a small circle of DNA called a plasmid, that can flit from one type of bacterium to another. A single plasmid can provide a slew of different resistances. In 1968, 12,500 people in Guatemala died in an epidemic of Shigella diarrhea. The microbe harbored a plasmid carrying resistances to four antibiotics!

A Vicious Cycle: More Infections and Antibiotic Overuse

Though bacterial antibiotic resistance is a natural phenomenon, societal factors also contribute to the problem. These factors include increased infection transmission, coupled with inappropriate antibiotic use.

More people are contracting infections. Sinusitis among adults is on the rise, as are ear infections in children. A report by CDC's Linda F. McCaig and James M. Hughes, M.D., in the Jan. 18, 1995, Journal of the American Medical Association, tracks antibiotic use in treating common illnesses. The report cites nearly 6 million antibiotic prescriptions for sinusitis in 1985, and nearly 13 million in 1992. Similarly, for middle ear infections, the numbers are 15 million prescriptions in 1985, and 23.6 million in 1992.

Causes for the increase in reported infections are diverse. Some studies correlate the doubling in doctor's office visits for ear infections for preschoolers between 1975 and 1990 to increased use of day-care facilities. Homelessness contributes to the spread of infection. Ironically, advances in modern medicine have made more people predisposed to infection. People on chemotherapy and transplant recipients taking drugs to suppress their immune function are at greater risk of infection.

"There are the number of immunocompromised patients, who wouldn't have survived in earlier times," says Cranston. "Radical procedures produce patients who are in difficult shape in the hospital, and are prone to nosocomial [hospital-acquired] infections. Also, the general aging of patients who live longer, get sicker, and die slower contributes to the problem," he adds.

Though some people clearly need to be treated with antibiotics, many experts are concerned about the inappropriate use of these powerful drugs. "Many consumers have an expectation that when they're ill, antibiotics are the answer. They put pressure on the physician to prescribe them. Most of the time the illness is viral, and antibiotics are not the answer. This large burden of antibiotics is certainly selecting resistant bacteria," says Blum.

Another much-publicized concern is use of antibiotics in livestock, where the drugs are used in well animals to prevent disease, and the animals are later slaughtered for food. "If an animal gets a bacterial infection, growth is slowed and it doesn't put on weight as fast," says Joe Madden, Ph.D., strategic manager of microbiology at FDA's Center for Food Safety and Applied Nutrition. In addition, antibiotics are sometimes administered at low levels in feed for long durations to increase the rate of weight gain and improve the efficiency of converting animal feed to units of animal production.

FDA's Center for Veterinary Medicine limits the amount of antibiotic residue in poultry and other meats, and the U.S. Department of Agriculture monitors meats for drug residues. According to Margaret Miller, Ph.D., deputy division director at the Center for Veterinary Medicine, the residue limits for antimicrobial animal drugs are set low enough to ensure that the residues themselves do not select resistant bacteria in (human) gut flora.

FDA is investigating whether bacteria resistant to quinolone antibiotics can emerge in food animals and cause disease in humans. Although thorough cooking sharply reduces the likelihood of antibiotic-resistant bacteria surviving in a meat meal to infect a human, it could happen.

Pathogens resistant to drugs other than fluoroquinolones have sporadically been reported to survive in a meat meal to infect a human. In 1983, for example, 18 people in four midwestern states developed multi-drug-resistant Salmonella food poisoning after eating beef from cows fed antibiotics. Eleven of the people were hospitalized, and one died. A study conducted by Alain Cometta, M.D., and his colleagues at the Centre Hospitalier Universitaire Vaudois in Lausanne, Switzerland, and reported in the April 28, 1994, New England Journal of Medicine, showed that increase in antibiotic resistance parallels increase in antibiotic use in humans. They examined a large group of cancer patients given antibiotics called fluoroquinolones to prevent infection. The patients' white blood cell counts were very low as a result of their cancer treatment, leaving them open to infection.

Between 1983 and 1993, the percentage of such patients receiving antibiotics rose from 1.4 to 45. During those years, the researchers isolated Escherichia coli bacteria annually from the patients, and tested the microbes for resistance to five types of fluoroquinolones. Between 1983 and 1990, all 92 E. coli strains tested were easily killed by the antibiotics. But from 1991 to 1993, 11 of 40 tested strains (28 percent) were resistant to all five drugs.

Towards Solving the Problem

Antibiotic resistance is inevitable, say scientists, but there are measures we can take to slow it. Efforts are under way on several fronts--improving infection control, developing new antibiotics, and using drugs more appropriately.

Barbara E. Murray, M.D., of the University of Texas Medical School at Houston writes in the April 28, 1994, New England Journal of Medicine that simple improvements in public health measures can go a long way towards preventing infection. Such approaches include more frequent hand washing by health-care workers, quick identification and isolation of patients with drug-resistant infections, and improving sewage systems and water purity in developing nations.

Drug manufacturers are once again becoming interested in developing new antibiotics. These efforts have been spurred both by the appearance of new bacterial illnesses, such as Lyme disease and Legionnaire's disease, and resurgences of old foes, such as tuberculosis, due to drug resistance.

FDA is doing all it can to speed development and availability of new antibiotic drugs. "We can't identify new agents--that's the job of the pharmaceutical industry. But once they have identified a promising new drug for resistant infections, what we can do is to meet with the company very early and help design the development plan and clinical trials," says Blum. In addition, drugs in development can be used for patients with multi-drug-resistant infections on an "emergency IND (compassionate use)" basis, if the physician requests this of FDA, Blum adds. This is done for people with AIDS or cancer, for example.

No one really has a good idea of the extent of antibiotic resistance, because it hasn't been monitored in a coordinated fashion. "Each hospital monitors its own resistance, but there is no good national system to test for antibiotic resistance," says Blum.

This may soon change. CDC is encouraging local health officials to track resistance data, and the World Health Organization has initiated a global computer database for physicians to report outbreaks of drug-resistant bacterial infections.

Experts agree that antibiotics should be restricted to patients who can truly benefit from them--that is, people with bacterial infections. Already this is being done in the hospital setting, where the routine use of antibiotics to prevent infection in certain surgical patients is being reexamined.

"We have known since way back in the antibiotic era that these drugs have been used inappropriately in surgical prophylaxis [preventing infections in surgical patients]. But there is more success [in limiting antibiotic use] in hospital settings, where guidelines are established, than in the more typical outpatient settings," says Cranston.

Murray points out an example of antibiotic prophylaxis in the outpatient setting--children with recurrent ear infections given extended antibiotic prescriptions to prevent future infections. (See "Protecting Little Pitchers' Ears" in the December 1994 FDA Consumer.)

Another problem with antibiotic use is that patients often stop taking the drug too soon, because symptoms improve. However, this merely encourages resistant microbes to proliferate. The infection returns a few weeks later, and this time a different drug must be used to treat it.

Targeting TB

Stephen Weis and colleagues at the University of North Texas Health Science Center in Fort Worth reported in the April 28, 1994, New England Journal of Medicine on research they conducted in Tarrant County, Texas, that vividly illustrates how helping patients to take the full course of their medication can actually lower resistance rates. The subject--tuberculosis.

TB is an infection that has experienced spectacular ups and downs. Drugs were developed to treat it, complacency set in that it was beaten, and the disease resurged because patients stopped their medication too soon and infected others. Today, one in seven new TB cases is resistant to the two drugs most commonly used to treat it (isoniazid and rifampin), and 5 percent of these patients die.

In the Texas study, 407 patients from 1980 to 1986 were allowed to take their medication on their own. From 1986 until the end of 1992, 581 patients were closely followed, with nurses observing them take their pills. By the end of the study, the relapse rate--which reflects antibiotic resistance--fell from 20.9 to 5.5 percent. This trend is especially significant, the researchers note, because it occurred as risk factors for spreading TB--including AIDS, intravenous drug use, and homelessness--were increasing.

The conclusion: Resistance can be slowed if patients take medications correctly.

Narrowing the Spectrum

Appropriate prescribing also means that physicians use "narrow spectrum" antibiotics--those that target only a few bacterial types--whenever possible, so that resistances can be restricted. The only national survey of antibiotic prescribing practices of office physicians, conducted by the National Center for Health Statistics, finds that the number of prescriptions has not risen appreciably from 1980 to 1992, but there has been a shift to using costlier, broader spectrum agents. This prescribing trend heightens the resistance problem, write McCaig and Hughes, because more diverse bacteria are being exposed to antibiotics.

One way FDA can help physicians choose narrower spectrum antibiotics is to ensure that labeling keeps up with evolving bacterial resistances. Blum hopes that the surveillance information on emerging antibiotic resistances from CDC will enable FDA to require that product labels be updated with the most current surveillance information.

Many of us have come to take antibiotics for granted. A child develops strep throat or an ear infection, and soon a bottle of "pink medicine" makes everything better. An adult suffers a sinus headache, and antibiotic pills quickly control it.

But infections can and do still kill. Because of a complex combination of factors, serious infections may be on the rise. While awaiting the next "wonder drug," we must appreciate, and use correctly, the ones that we already have.

Big Difference

If this bacterium could be shown four times bigger, it would be the right relative size to the virus beneath it. (Both are microscopic and are shown many times larger than life.)

Although bacteria are single-celled organisms, viruses are far simpler, consisting of one type of biochemical (a nucleic acid, such as DNA or RNA) wrapped in another (protein). Most bi-ologists do not consider viruses to be living things, but instead, infectious particles. Antibiotic drugs attack bacteria, not viruses.

Vancomycin Resistance Crisis

When microbes began resisting penicillin, medical researchers fought back with chemical cousins, such as methicillin and oxacillin. By 1953, the